Natural Hazard Mitigation Policy

About the Series

Recent years have shown that all manner of disasters have become increasingly damaging, dangerous and complex. Recent examples include the 2004 South Asian tsunami, Hurricane Katrina in 2005, and the Sichuan earthquake of 2008.

Disasters like these have, for years, been understood as neither strictly man-made or strictly natural; most disasters are a complex blend physical forces and social organization. And some disasters, such as the Madrid bombings of 2004 and the London bombings of 2005, are man-made, but their effects are vast, with structural, social, and environmental ramifications that reverberate locally, nationally, and globally. We cannot explain the full complexity of these events using single-discipline approaches.

This series will therefore reflect and promote the increasingly interdisciplinary nature of hazards and disaster research. Its reach will be wide because hazards research is very broad, encompassing such varied fields of study as research on industrial accidents, research on public health, biosecurity issues and "homeland security", just to name a few. And its reach will include an wide array of facets because scholars from the social, natural, and behavioral sciences have concluded that we cannot fully understand hazards and disasters without an appreciation for the social, natural and man-made environments involved.

In addressing the technical, social and environmental issues of hazards and disasters, this series will include up-to-date, comprehensive texts on key hazards and disasters at the local, regional, national, and global levels. It will cover numerous issues critical to successful research and practice and will consider these issues through an international lens. And it will involve all fields connected to the study of hazards and natural disasters, including disciplines found within the natural sciences, physical sciences, social sciences, and engineering. The series' coverage will therefore be broad, but it will be centered on the interactions between society, technology, and the natural environment in the hazards and disasters field.

Proposals for this book series may be sent to the Series Editor, Thomas A. Birkland, Kretzer Professor of Public Policy, North Carolina State University, at tom_birkland@ncsu.edu or the Publishing Editor, Tamara Welschot, at Tamara.Welschot@springer.com

Editorial Board:

For further volumes:
http://www.springer.com/series/8583

Daniel J. Alesch • Lucy A. Arendt
William J. Petak

Natural Hazard Mitigation Policy

Implementation, Organizational Choice, and Contextual Dynamics

Springer

Dr. Daniel J. Alesch
University of Wisconsin-Green Bay
WI, USA
djalesch@att.net

Lucy A. Arendt
University of Wisconsin-Green Bay
WI, USA
ArendtL@uwgb.edu

William J. Petak
University of Southern California
Los Angeles
CA, USA
petak@usc.edu

This work was supported primarily by the Earthquake Engineering Research Centers Program of the National Science Foundation under NSF Award Number EEC-9701471 to the Multidisciplinary Center for Earthquake Engineering Research. Any opinions, findings and conclusions or recommendations expressed in this material are those of the authors and do not necessarily reflect those of the National Science Foundation.

ISBN 978-94-007-2234-7 e-ISBN 978-94-007-2235-4
DOI 10.1007/978-94-007-2235-4
Springer Dordrecht Heidelberg London New York

Library of Congress Control Number: 2011939300

Printed on acid-free paper

Springer is part of Springer Science+Business Media (www.springer.com)

Preface

This book is fundamentally about implementing public policy intended to mitigate the consequences stemming from hazardous events, particularly extreme natural hazard events. More than that, it focuses on the importance, when formulating public policy, of understanding the problem at hand in its various dimensions and from various perspectives, the importance of devising policies and programs based on an understanding of the likely consequences of implementing them, and the importance of taking steps to reduce the frequency and impact of adverse unanticipated consequences stemming from implementation.

Working together over the years, we have come to some basic, mutually shared conclusions. We have become convinced that, if one is to understand policy implementation, it is necessary to look beyond what government administrators do or do not do and the complexities of administration when many agencies at various levels of government are involved. One must look at the assumptions of cause and effect underlying the design of the policy itself, the anticipated responses of targeted populations, and the likelihood that things might not work out as anticipated. Years ago, we may have been surprised when things did not work out as expected; now, we are equally as surprised when things do work out as expected. It is essential to understand how the environment within which a policy is being administered affects the outcomes of attempting to administer the policy. Chance events confound policies based on relative certainty about "if we do this, then that will happen." The relevancy and the efficacy of policies change as the context within which they are promulgated changes. The relative long-term success of public policy design and implementation depends on the entire context within which the process takes place. As the context changes, so too must the policy. Rigidity in policy making and implementation limits the capacity of the affected system to achieve the initially desired outcomes in the face of dynamic contextual change.

In the case study that is the focus of this book, neither of the key stakeholder groups emerges clearly as the "good guy" or the "bad guy." Advocates of seismic safety sincerely believe that they are doing the right thing. Hospital administrators, charged with responding to what they call "an unfunded legislative mandate," also sincerely believe that they are doing the right thing. We have concluded that both are right in their perceptions of themselves, though perhaps not right in finding a mutually acceptable way forward. Our perception that both advocates and opponents are sincere has already caused some of our colleagues to tell us that we favor one side over the other. That simply isn't the case.

How can both sets of stakeholders be right? Two authors help us to understand this phenomenon. One of these authors, Harold Lasswell, a noted political scientist, observed that people are generally rational, but that they are typically rational to any one or any mix of different value bases. One person might be rational to the base "equity" while another person might be rational to the base "economic efficiency." When the two individuals look at a particular set of phenomena, they interpret the implications differently and, thus, hold different opinions concerning the phenomena. The second author is also a noted observer of human behavior. Kurt Vonnegut in a little known novel, "The Sirens of Titan," discusses a phenomenon of his own invention called the "chronosynclastic infundibulum." For Vonnegut, one of these phenomena exists between earth and Mars. It is a place in which the differences between completely opposite viewpoints concerning some matter are inherently resolved. In brief, two people can look at the same phenomenon, see it very differently, and both be right. The secret to progress is acknowledging this possibility, and then looking for a shared understanding that enables movement forward.

We have pointed out how important we perceive chance events to be in the course of events. This book itself is the outcome of chance events. Half a century ago, in the late 1960s, two of this book's authors, Dan Alesch and Bill Petak, along with Art Atkisson, became acquainted when they were at the School of Public Administration at the University of Southern California (USC). At the time, each was pursuing slightly different activities. Bill was heavily into public systems management, Art was heading an institute on urban ecology, and Dan was working on designing computer-driven information and decision support systems for local government applications. Bill became a member of the USC faculty in systems management and public administration, Art moved to the University of Houston, and Dan joined the Rand Corporation. About a decade later, Art and Dan found each other again in Green Bay, Wisconsin, where Art had accepted an offer to create a program in public and environmental administration at the brand new University of Wisconsin-Green Bay. Dan had moved to Green Bay for Rand to administer site operations for a large housing assistance experiment. Before long, the three were back working together on natural hazard concerns. Bill and Art were completing a major book, 'Natural Hazard Risk Assessment and Public Policy: Anticipating the Unexpected," and, as the Rand project wound down, Art had convinced Dan to join him on the faculty at UW-Green Bay.

Despite the subtitle of the book Bill and Art had published, we don't always anticipate the unexpected. Art, a very dear friend and colleague, died unexpectedly midway through an NSF-funded project he and Bill were conducting, having to do with mitigating the earthquake hazard associated with unreinforced masonry buildings. So, more than 30 years ago, Bill Petak and Dan Alesch undertook the completion of that project. The outcome of that effort was a book entitled "The Politics and Economics of Earthquake Hazard Mitigation." That book examined the decades of difficulty and frustration that the cities of Long Beach and Los Angeles experienced while trying to get owners to either enhance the seismic resistance of their unreinforced masonry buildings or to demolish them. We concluded that a primary reason it took so long and was so difficult to accomplish the goal was because the local governments failed to look at the problem from the perspective of the owners and to devise policies that would accommodate their basic needs, as well as those of the city governments. Ultimately, policymakers did just that and the problem of old unreinforced masonry buildings began to be greatly diminished.

Over the years, Bill and Dan continued to work together on projects related to natural hazards and mitigation. In the 1990s, Bill invited Dan to join him in conducting an analysis of implementation problems related to California legislation requiring that old hospital facilities in California be retrofitted to enhance seismic resistance, be replaced, or be removed from use as acute care facilities. Bill, while at USC, was a member of the Multidisciplinary Center for Earthquake Engineering Research (MCEER) research team working on projects initiated by an NSF-supported national earthquake center housed in the University at Buffalo, one of the SUNY campuses. A representative of the California Office of Statewide Health Planning and Development, Chris Tokas, served on MCEER's external board of advisors and suggested that MCEER conduct a study of the implementation of a new law, SB 1953, recently enacted by California to address pre-1973 acute care hospital facilities that did not meet contemporary standards for seismic resistance. MCEER agreed and Bill was selected to head the study. He subsequently asked Dan to work with him, and the project resulting in this book was born.

It didn't take very long in the analysis for them to understand that the decisions being made by the hospitals subject to the new public policy were critical to what was happening with program implementation. Fortunately for us and for the hazards field of study, when Dan approached Lucy Arendt about joining the research team, she agreed to do so. Lucy is an associate professor of management in the Cofrin School of Business at the University of Wisconsin-Green Bay with a focus on organizational behavior and decision making. She instantly became a full-fledged member of the team, bringing fresh eyes and important insights to the project. With Lucy becoming a full-fledged member of the team, with Dan a formally educated political economist, and Bill an engineer who moved on to public systems management, the combined efforts and approach to the study of SB 1953 policy implementation became very much an interdisciplinary effort.

The result of this long-standing collaboration is the book that you are about to read.

Acknowledgements

We are grateful to the hundreds of people with whom we have spoken on matters related to SB 1953 over the past decade on the condition of their anonymity: public officials, hospital owners and administrators, structural engineers, and professionals in related fields with an interest in the policy and its outcomes. We are grateful to scholars and practitioners who read early drafts of our material and commented on them with considerable perspicacity. We extend our special thanks to J. and B., William Anderson, and Peter May.

This work was supported in large part by the Earthquake Engineering Research Centers Program of the National Science Foundation under NSF Award Number EEC-9701471 to the Multidisciplinary Center for Earthquake Engineering Research (MCEER). The Center, with NSF funds, supported a very considerable proportion of our field research and early reports. Without the financial support from NSF and MCEER, this research could not have been conducted. We are particularly appreciative to the management and staff of MCEER who supported our work, including Michel Bruneau, Andre Filiatrault, George Lee, Jane Stoyle Welch, Sofia A. Tangalos, and all the members of the current and past support staff. Any opinions, findings and conclusions or recommendations expressed in this material are those of the authors and do not necessarily reflect those of either the National Science Foundation or MCEER.

Last, but certainly not least, we extend our deepest appreciation to our respective spouses and families for their support over the decade or so during which this activity has had us travelling across California, the West Coast and the Gulf Coast, sitting at a computer or in a chair reading for hours on end while oblivious to most other things, and rambling on almost endlessly at inappropriate times about matters relating to the nexus of public policy formation and implementation, organizational decision making, earthquakes, and hospitals.

Green Bay, Wisconsin — Daniel J. Alesch
Green Bay, Wisconsin — Lucy A. Arendt
Rancho Palos Verdes, California — William J. Petak

Contents

Chapter 1
The Starting Point: A Confluence of Questions About Policy Design and Implementation

1.1 The Problem

Few things are as simple as they first appear.

The consequences of natural hazard events are large, pervasive, expensive, and growing. At the same time, implementing public regulatory policy to reduce the consequences of those events is rarely as straightforward or as successful as one might think. Neither the consequences of natural hazard events nor the continuing problems associated with implementing public policies to reduce those consequences is a trivial matter. This book focuses on gaining a greater understanding of public policy implementation, particularly as it applies to regulatory policy aimed at reducing the likely consequences of natural hazard events.

Newcomers to government often assume that a policy, once adopted, will be implemented faithfully in accord with the policymakers' intent and have the desired results. An increasingly rich body of research confirms what old hands already know: That is simply not the case.

Policies usually, either implicitly or explicitly, identify at least the general means by which they are to be implemented. When the agency that is specified in a policy directive begins to design the program and outline the regulations that define the policy in operational terms, implementation begins in earnest. This period can easily involve as much political interplay as did the process of enacting the legislation. Practitioners and scholars alike have come to understand that policy adoption is simply one milestone in an ongoing process of policy development. Calista's (1994) assessment is that the field of study has evolved from one of viewing implementation as simply the process of carrying out policy directives to one where implementation is now integral to the field of policy intervention, including recognizing its influence on policy formulation.

The reality is that policy may or may not be implemented as envisaged by those who put the policy in place. During implementation, policy may be altered or adapted either intentionally or inadvertently. The extent to which a policy leads to

D.J. Alesch et al., *Natural Hazard Mitigation Policy: Implementation, Organizational Choice, and Contextual Dynamics*, Environmental Hazards,
DOI 10.1007/978-94-007-2235 4_1, © Springer Science+Business Media B.V. 2012

the intended outcomes depends on many variables, only some of which may be controlled by policy makers. Moreover, policies often have significant, unanticipated consequences during implementation that may need to be addressed in order to move forward. Again, few things are as simple as they appear.

Multiple stakeholders, with varying perspectives, over time, and with differential access to information and resources – all tend to add complexity to what might seem to be straightforward and even simple prescriptions, goals, and preferred actions. Case in point: One might say that hospitals and other critical buildings like schools should remain standing and functional after an earthquake. Hospital patients and workers, schoolchildren and teachers – all should feel safe when faced with a natural hazard event such as an earthquake. Setting these simple statements aside, the reality of making them happen is complicated, and the path to goal achievement is seldom obvious. Different stakeholders interpret goal statements differently, have different values, change their views over time, and may or may not have the information and resources to achieve goals, regardless of the support those goals may have engendered.

This book explores the case of a state government regulatory effort to strengthen California's inventory of acute care hospital buildings against earthquakes. The effort is known as SB 1953. The case is a story of well-meaning seismic safety advocates attempting to require equally well-intentioned hospital owners and operators to retrofit acute care facilities built before 1973 to meet contemporary seismic standards, to replace them, or to remove them from service. The case is fraught with complexity. Nothing is simple. Neither the independent elements, nor the interdependent relationships, are easily understood.

1.2 Hazard Policy Implementation: Not a Trivial Concern

The consequences of natural and manmade hazard events are anything but trivial. Worldwide in 2010, for example, nearly 260,000 people perished in natural and man-made disasters, insured losses for the global insurance industry were more than $36 billion, and direct economic losses were in excess of $222 billion (Greil 2010). Each year, massive amounts of uninsured losses are borne by property owners, including extraordinary and uncounted costs of persistent community economic and social consequences stemming from the event. Perhaps even more importantly, the people affected have to bear the extraordinary emotional and psychological costs of being displaced from their homes or communities, from injury and death to loved ones, and from having their hopes and dreams shattered.

The problem isn't going away. Direct losses from hazard events and the consequences that cascade in their aftermath are astonishingly high now, and they are growing, as the most rapid population growth in the United States is taking place in locations that are inherently dangerous and as people and organizations fail to take adequate precautions. Despite the extraordinary social and economic costs of hazard events, Americans expend relatively little money and effort to reduce the likely consequences of hazards on themselves, those they love, and their organizations.

One could argue that we are optimists who believe that bad things won't happen or that we'll be able to repair whatever damage occurs. Or, one could say that we expect the government (local, state, and federal) to "make us whole" if we suffer losses. Perhaps we see that as our due as taxpayers. Or, one could say that we live in the moment, and prefer not to dwell on possible future outcomes. No matter what one says, it's clear that Americans are often ill prepared for hazard events and their consequences, especially outlier or extreme events that may include two or more disasters. A good example of an extreme event occurred in 2005, when Hurricane Katrina struck New Orleans, Louisiana. While the hurricane itself caused relatively little damage to the built environment, the flooding that swamped 80% of New Orleans in the aftermath of Katrina was devastating to not only the built environment, but also to the natural, social, and economic environments of New Orleans. Nearly 6 years later, New Orleans is still not recovered.

In addition to the costs incurred because of hazard events at home, Americans contribute massive amounts of money and material to those who suffer in disasters in other nations. Uncounted amounts of assistance flowed from the United States to those who suffered from the massive 2004 Indian Ocean Tsunami that killed almost 300,000 people, the devastating Haitian and Chilean earthquakes in 2010, and the tragic earthquake and tsunami that wreaked havoc on the northeast coast of Japan in early 2011. United States citizens are willing to help in the face of disaster, and we are supported in these efforts through tax credits and other mechanisms.

Scientists have sufficient understanding and engineers have sufficient technology to enable us to reduce substantially injuries and loss of life as well as damage to the built environment from most of the disasters experienced in the United States each year. That is not to say that we have the ability to protect ourselves completely from truly rare and devastating events such as Earth's collision with a large asteroid some 65 million years ago, the volcanic eruption that buried Pompeii and Herculaneum in 79, the 2004 Indian Ocean Tsunami, the Richter 8.8 earthquake in Chile in 2010, or the Richter 9.0 earthquake in Japan in 2011. We have the technical means, however, to reduce losses substantially from the most frequent and typical hurricanes, floods, earthquakes, tornadoes, winter storms, and other hazardous events we experience. We also have the technology to reduce the consequences of terrorist attacks from domestic and foreign interests.

In response to what they perceive to be inadequate preparations, advocates for enhanced safety from hazard events continue to work hard to get legislative bodies to adopt hazard mitigation policies into law and, then, convert them into programs that are intended to induce individuals and organizations to take additional precautions. These policies are not advocated by "busybody do-gooders" who want to dictate the personal behavior of others. Typically, advocates for hazard mitigation hold that, when private action or inaction creates considerable potential for losses not only to knowing risk takers, but also to the community at large, government has the right and, indeed, the obligation to take action in an attempt to alter that risky behavior. Consequently, governments have enacted policies to regulate land use, building construction, traffic and driving, and a host of other matters. History shows, however, that good intentions do not always result in good legislation, nor does good legislation always result in effective programs. Program implementation often takes longer than expected, has unexpected consequences, and costs much more than anticipated.

Calista (1994) tells us that, at the simplest level, implementation represents the faithful fulfillment of policy intentions by public servants. Newcomers to business and government often assume that a policy, once adopted, will be implemented in accord with the policymakers' intent. For better or worse, this is not always the case.

The nominal regulatory policy process comprises policy, implementation, outputs, and outcomes. Authorized individuals or bodies make policy in response to some perceived problem. Authorized agents are responsible for implementing the policy. Implementation results in program output and those outputs modify the targeted population, leading to outcomes. This straightforward, linear, and even rational process assumes shared perceptions and goals, plentiful and accurate information, and stakeholders' ability to manage and act upon information irrespective of their personal interests. But, then, the nominal case is usually a generalization that masks the fact that nothing is as simple as it first appears. And, assumptions that people are rational decision makers may be unfounded.

Practitioners and scholars have come to understand that policy adoption is simply one milestone in a continuing process of addressing an issue. It may be that successful implementation of the intent of the policy is the exception rather than the rule. Calista reports that the most prevalent finding in implementation research is that outcomes are either disappointing or unwitting (Calista 1994). Burby and colleagues (1998) report that research demonstrates severe slippage in compliance with rules promulgated by planners and code-writing agencies. The U. S. Office of Technology Assessment refers to what it calls an "implementation gap." Illustrating this gap, although many communities, especially in California, have taken steps to mitigate earthquake losses, there remains a significant difference between what current knowledge says can be done and what actually gets done. The Office of Technology Assessment opined that the National Earthquake Hazard Reduction Program's greatest challenge is addressing the implementation gap (Office of Technology Assessment 1995).

1.3 Three Critical Questions

The intent of our research is to develop insights into three fundamental and tightly interrelated questions concerning public policy implementation, particularly implementation of public regulatory policy focused on mitigating the consequences of hazardous events. Answers to these questions are central to reducing the likely consequences of hazardous events, including especially extreme events, willful and mindless acts of destruction, major accidents, and pandemics on individuals, organizations, and communities. The three questions are:

1. What are the primary obstacles to implementing public regulatory policies intended to reduce the risks associated with hazardous events?

2. How do formal organizations make choices about how much if anything to spend to mitigate the likely consequences of rare but potential extremely destructive events?
3. What characteristics of public policies intended to reduce the risks associated with hazardous events increase the likelihood that those policies will be implemented successfully?

The implementation problem is not unique to policies aimed at mitigating the potential adverse consequences of hazardous events; it is widespread among areas of public concern. The three fundamental questions essentially constitute three interwoven threads that comprise the dominant pattern of the fabric making up this case study of public regulatory policy implementation. That fabric incorporates elements of problem framing and sensemaking, special interest group roles in policy making, organizational behavior and decision making in the face of considerable uncertainty, public policy design, legislative behavior, political behavior, and the impact of contextual dynamics on program outcomes. All together, they make up what we call the *ecology of public policy implementation.*

1.3.1 Obstacles to Policy Implementation

The first fundamental question has to do with obstacles to implementing policies and programs successfully. As noted in the introductory paragraphs, scholarly research focused on policy and program implementation demonstrates conclusively that successful implementation does not follow policy adoption as night follows day. This might be particularly true in the case of policies aimed at reducing the adverse consequences of hazardous events, especially when the public policy calls for organizations other than the policy making government to bear the expense of doing so. The case we have studied over more than a decade has provided an excellent opportunity for us to build upon the existing body of literature having to do with obstacles to policy implementation.

Policy implementation lags far behind advances in scientific and technical understanding. Perhaps that is because comparatively little attention has been focused on the question of how to improve implementation. An inadequate understanding exists of how to overcome barriers and disincentives associated with implementing hazard mitigation policy. Our research is based on the premise that understanding the context of and obstacles to implementation might inform us as to how we might improve the likelihood that risk reduction measures against hazardous events will be implemented. We examine why organizations take or fail to take precautions and what might be done to increase significantly the proportion of them that do act to reduce losses to life and property from natural hazards, specifically earthquakes.

Although the focus of the book is on implementing policy intended to reduce the adverse consequences of hazardous events, especially extreme events, we believe our findings have relevance and significance for policy and program design and implementation in many substantive areas of concern. Ultimately, we are interested in presenting an authentic assessment of the conditions under which public policy is most likely to be implemented as intended, while minimizing unintended and often undesirable consequences.

1.3.2 The Hazard Mitigation Investment Decision

The second fundamental question has to do with how formal organizations make what we call "the hazard mitigation investment decision." People who are deeply concerned with reducing the adverse consequences of hazardous events on communities, organizations, and individuals have come to realize that, just because people might understand the risks, it is often difficult to enact and then implement measures to reduce those risks. Advances in scientific understanding of the likely consequences of hazards and means for mitigating those consequences have far outstripped individual and collective action to reduce the consequences. Despite attempts by hazard safety advocates to demonstrate positive benefit-to-cost ratios of hazard mitigation, many organizations and individuals do not take steps to mitigate hazards even when methods for doing so exist.

Public policies often call for organizations outside the government making the policy to make, at their own expense, the investments necessary to achieve the policy objective. The organizations targeted by these policies often refer to such policies as "unfunded mandates." The response of the entities targeted by government policy to make investments or change behaviors is one that is extremely important, but that has been generally overlooked by those studying implementation. Hill suggests that it is understandable that this topic has been generally overlooked.

> . . . the focus of the traditional implementation and public administration literature lies mostly on governmental – or at least nominally governmentally controlled – entities. Implementation scholars are usually educated as political scientists, and as such they notice what they have been trained to see. But by ignoring nongovernmental actors in the implementation process, scholars have overlooked important factors that shape implementation . . . (2003 p. 268)

When formal organizations are presented with information about the likely impacts of hazardous events on them, they often fail to take actions to reduce the risk of significant losses from those events. Even when legislation mandates organizational or individual action to reduce risk, sometimes it is extremely difficult to compel the desired behavior on the part of others. A gap between knowing and doing exists (Pfeffer and Sutton 2000), and may be difficult to bridge. Multiple, often competing, priorities and demands on resources may interfere with organizations paying attention to infrequent events like earthquakes that may never cause substantial damage. Organizational leaders, by definition, are gamblers of a sort who must decide which risks are reasonable and which are not, and how to respond. These individuals do not expect to eliminate all risks so much as manage them.

Normative models exist to guide or assist organizations when faced with decisions about how much to invest in mitigating the consequences of possible calamities (e.g., expected present value of possible future losses, benefit-cost analysis), but we have come to believe that, in many cases, those models are not particularly informative or helpful to organizational leaders. Relatively little has been done to develop a descriptive model of how organizations actually make decisions about investing in hazard mitigation or risk reduction when confronted with multiple criteria and multiple objectives, especially when benefits and consequences are guesses or, at best, probability distributions with wide confidence intervals.

We believe this to be a critically important, but largely unexplored part of both the organizational decision making and the hazard mitigation literatures. Here, we examine how organizational decision makers frame and approach questions of what, if anything, to do about rare and unlikely hazardous events which, should they occur, may well spell ruin for the organization, particularly if steps are not taken beforehand to reduce their impacts. Our study of organizational decision making concerning hazard mitigation sheds light on that aspect of the obstacles to policy and program implementation.

Our intent is to lay out a framework for an empirically based understanding of how organizations frame the hazard mitigation problem and make choices about what, if anything, to do. That is, how do organizations decide how many, if any, of their resources they will apply to reducing the likely consequences of rare but potentially ruinous events on the organization or its constituents? Presumably, knowing how organizations frame the problem and make decisions about it will inform the development of authentic normative methods.

1.3.3 Improving the Design of Hazard Mitigation Policies to Enhance the Likelihood of Implementation

Our third and final fundamental question centers on how to devise hazard mitigation policies that are likely to result in the desired outcomes. We are interested in gaining greater understanding of the characteristics of public policy and programs that are likely to increase the probability that they will be implemented.

Creating sophisticated policy intended to serve the common good is necessary, but not sufficient, for implementing the policy and achieving the common good. Our purpose is to learn how to increase the probability that public policy, as expressed in statutes, codes, and ordinances, will be carried out consistent with legislative intent and, further, that the policy implementation results in the intended consequences.

If public policy is intended to result in people and organizations taking action to protect themselves and those around them, it is important to base those policies on an understanding of the obstacles to implementation and how individuals and organizations make hazard mitigation investment decisions. We need to understand what facilitates and drives action on the part of affected organizations and individuals.

1.4 Approaches to Understanding Implementation

1.4.1 *Emerging Perspectives*

Legislative or executive policies typically designate one or more governmental organizations to develop programs that result in money being spent, action being taken, and, presumably, changes in behavior. At the simplest level, implementation represents the faithful fulfillment of those policy intentions by public servants (Calista 1994). Beyond that basic description, however, there are significant differences of opinion of what constitutes implementation. One alternative view is that implementation analysis should include not only the outputs of agency activities and behaviors, but the outcomes of the policy, those activities, and other variables as well. That is, the analyst should look to see the extent to which the policy itself and its administration have contributed to the desired outcomes that gave rise to the policy.

Early studies of public policy implementation focused primarily on administrative behavior by government agencies and operatives. One of the very important contributions to our understanding of implementation stemming from the early studies of the role of administrative agencies in implementation is that policy development continues during implementation. Pressman and Wildavsky (1973), for example, focused on how the process proceeded when multiple agencies at various levels of government were engaged in program administration, including agency politics and behaviors, noting the importance of implementation behaviors on the policy itself. Lipsky (1971) says that successful implementation comes down to how "street level" administrators use their discretion to implement or not implement the policy. Lipsky goes further to suggest that control over implementation "goes to those who gain power over determining how worker discretion is defined and to those who determine how operation routines are changed" (cited in Calista 1994). Allison and Halperin (cited in Bardach 1977) agree. They suggest that new departures in policy stem from some decision by central players, but the specific details are determined in large part by standard operating procedure and programs existing in the organization at the time. Hill and Hupe make the point clearly:

> What can be called 'public policy', and thus has to be implemented, is the product of what has happened in the earlier stages of the policy process. Nevertheless, the content of that policy, and its impact on those affected, may be substantially modified, elaborated, or even negated during the implementation stage, as Anderson points out. "(P)olicy is made as it is being administered and administered as it is being made" (2002, p. 6).

Mazmanian and Sabatier (1989, pp. 7–9) address the matter of what constitutes implementation by discussing the elements of a process that involves policy formulation, implementation, and reformulation. Some scholars prefer to think of the three elements as clear and distinct from one another. It is true that the component parts of the process may be studied independently of one another, but Mazmanian and Sabatier suggest that they are also appropriately viewed as overlapping parts of a process that is often nonlinear, iterative, and muddled.

Increasingly, implementation analysts have expanded the appropriate analysis of implementation to include an analysis of the outcomes stemming from formulating and administering policy. Distinctions are made between the *outputs* of a policy or program and the *outcomes* resulting from the policy or program. This, according to Winter, is a fundamental issue about whether analysts should focus on implementation behavior or policy outcomes (cited in Hill and Hupe 2002, p. 146). Those who argue for focusing on administrative behavior or outputs arguably have the easier task. They can focus on how much of what was done without having to concern themselves with the consequences of external conditions or events that may affect outcomes. However, assessing the extent to which implementation is successful by relying on an analysis of administrative behavior and politics within and between government agencies is unlikely to help us understand fully why the specific outcomes stemming from a public policy implementation occur. Hill and Hupe (2002) point out that policy outcomes may be influenced by factors that have nothing to do with the intervention. Second, they suggest that judgments about outcomes may be influenced by factors that have nothing to do with the policy intervention. Third, outcome analysis suggests that system changes are likely to result in improved outcomes. Presumably, Hill and Hupe mean that the causal model underlying the intervention accurately depicts "what leads to what." Finally, Hill and Hupe argue that outcome analysis requires that one define "unambiguous and agreed outcome variables."

We, too, are concerned that a primary focus on what administrative agencies do in response to policy directives promulgates a view that public policy processes can be divided into discrete activities implying a linear process of policy making, policy implementation, policy reformulation, and outcomes that are tangent with one another but which do not interact and that are not iterative. Such a nominal case may be employed to help novices begin to gain an understanding of an extremely complex process, but, as we know, the nominal case is usually an abstraction masking the fact that nothing is as simple as it first appears. The actual case is one in which policy may be initiated by legislation, but in which policy may continue to be made by the administrators during implementation and in which the legislation itself may be revisited one or more times as outcomes occur or as those likely to be affected by the policy seek to alter it through legislative or administrative action. There is, of course, nothing inherently wrong with some analysts limiting their analysis to agency behaviors and outputs rather than outcomes. Those analyses have contributed to an improved understanding of organizational behavior as it relates to policy administration. Focusing on outputs rather than outcomes, however, answers only one set of questions and leaves other critically important questions unanswered.

Mazmanian and Sabatier (1989) state that the implementation process "normally runs through a number of stages." These begin "with passage of the basic statute, followed by the policy inputs (decisions) of the implementing agencies, the compliance of target groups with those decisions, the actual impacts – both intended and unintended – of those outputs, the perceived impacts of agency decisions, and finally, important revisions (or attempted revisions) in the basic statute" (pp. 20–21). In so saying, Mazmanian and Sabatier extend the concept of what comprises implementation to include three considerations beyond Calista's description of the simplest case. First, they include compliance of target groups (outcomes) with the policy as a key element of administration. Second, they include the intended and unintended consequences of policy and administration. Third, they include actual and attempted revisions to the basic enabling legislation.

Mazmanian and Sabatier (1989) add yet another set of considerations for those studying the implementation process. Specifically, they suggest that "the crucial role of implementation analysis is the identification of the variables which affect the achievement of legal objectives through this entire process" (pp. 20–21).

We understand from the literature that implementation is not subsequent to policy making, but, instead, an inherent part of it. Consequently, implementation must be as inherently political as policy making. The political aspects of implementation are probably essential and inevitable. Policies are continually redefined from formulation through implementation and, then, often back around the cycle again. Wildavsky (cited in Calista 1994) suggests that one reason is that "desirable policies are rarely self-evident." Calista goes on to suggest that implementation outcomes appear slowly and unevenly; continual adjustments, therefore, presumably make sense. Implementation, Calista (1994) suggests, is a gradualist phenomena. As a consequence, students of policy implementation have reflected on how policy changes in implementation. Majone and Wildavsky (1978) say policy choices *evolve*. Berman (1980) says policy choices *adapt*. Rein and Rabinowitz (1978) say policy choices *drift*. Whether they evolve, adapt, or drift, what's clear is that policy continues to be developed during implementation. The stages are not discrete.

One final point is particularly important. Those who administer policy are often involved directly in the policymaking process. Specifically, legislatures adopt policy statements that, typically, have the force of law. The operational policy, however, is almost always stated in the regulations devised by the lead administering agency and approved, subsequently, by the legislature or some authoritative agency within the executive branch. These administrative regulations become administrative law and form the total policy. For ease of understanding, in this book, when we talk about policy, we include both the bill enacted by the legislature or the policy directive issued by the executive *and* the administrative rules devised subsequently that govern the specifics of the policy.

1.4.2 Our Perspective

How one defines the appropriate focus of public policy implementation and research on policy implementation is critical. For our purposes, it is appropriate, indeed essential, that we take the broader perspective recommended by Mazmanian and Sabatier. We also believe it is important to distinguish between simple administration and implementation. Calista's (1994) description of implementation at the simplest level, we would argue, is simply administration, i.e., doing what one has been directed to do in the way one has been directed to do it, and doing so largely without regard to external consequences that may result. Implementation, we contend, includes administration by designated and authorized parties in government, but also extends to include the actions of those charged with conducting or mandated to conduct activities intended to result in the outcomes envisaged in the policy, regardless of whether they are governmental entities.

A final characteristic of our perspective is critically important. We believe that understanding context and contextual dynamics are of major importance when attempting to understand implementation of a particular public policy or cluster of public policies. Certainly, examining phenomena in the context of change is not a new concept; it has, we think, been omitted from much of the study of policy implementation. Contextual dynamics underlies much of the content in Gunderson and Holling's Panarchy: Understanding Transformations in Human and Natural Systems (Gunderson and Holling 2002). Contextual dynamics also play a central role in understanding how the case study that follows in this book plays out.

1.5 The Case Study

This book is based on the authors' case study of SB 1953, legislation enacted by the State of California and intended to improve the seismic resistance of older acute care hospital facilities in that state. The lessons from the case study are not unique to earthquakes and hospitals. They apply directly to other natural hazard regulatory policies and to policies intended to reduce the likelihood of adverse consequences of hazardous events generally. Beyond that, they can apply to problems endemic to implementing a wide range of public policies, including environmental issues, public health and safety, market regulation to ensure a well-functioning national economy, and, indeed, to other public policies intended to change the behavior of individuals or organizations to enhance the well-being of the public.

The case that serves as the focal point of this book illustrates well the fundamental axiom that few things are as simple as they appear. The case concerns mandated retrofitting, replacing, or withdrawing from use as acute care facilities older acute care hospital buildings in California – earthquake country. In considering the case, we are interested in better exploring and understanding the regulatory policy development and implementation process, as seen through the eyes of multiple key stakeholders. The stakeholders in the case are knowledgeable individuals representing their own and broader interests. They look at the same problem – making acute care hospital buildings safer from earthquakes – and see something different. We see our task as one of unraveling the various perspectives and interpreting the effect of, and the impact on, the regulatory policy process that engaged the different stakeholders in our focal case.

The study describes and examines a policy that was promulgated, ultimately, because of two major earthquakes in the Los Angeles, California, area. The first of these is the 1971 Sylmar Earthquake with an epicenter in the San Fernando Valley. That temblor resulted in the collapse of an unreinforced masonry building housing the Veterans Administration Hospital in San Fernando, killing 49 people. In the same event, the Olive View Hospital in Sylmar, which had opened just a month before the earthquake, suffered extensive damage. A two-story building became a one-story building as the first floor "soft story" collapsed. The main tower was so badly damaged that it could not be repaired. One person was killed as a portico covering an ambulance entrance collapsed, but no one inside the hospital was killed. Nonetheless, it took many years to build a new replacement hospital.

The failure of this new hospital may have been the prime impetus for the Alquist Hospital Facilities Act of 1972 because it represented the failure of the existing code, enforced by local agencies, to provide a brand new hospital that could remain functional after a major seismic event. The Act incorporated tougher design and construction standards for hospitals with the specific intent of reducing the likely adverse consequences of future earthquakes on hospitals. *Importantly, however, the Act did not require any changes to hospital buildings built prior to its enactment.*

About two decades later, in January 1994, the Northridge Earthquake, also centered in the San Fernando Valley, significantly damaged structures both in the Valley and in nearby portions of Los Angeles, Santa Monica, and other locales. Damage to acute care hospitals was of particular concern. At the time of the 1994 Northridge Earthquake, many hospital buildings built before 1973 were still being used for acute care delivery. While these acute care buildings were being withdrawn from the inventory more slowly than seismic safety advocates had anticipated and hoped, newer buildings tended to serve diagnostic and treatment purposes. Eight hospitals evacuated patients (Schultz et al. 2003) and many others incurred serious damage to structural building components and to nonstructural components within their buildings, limiting the buildings' ability to perform their intended functions following the earthquake. The hospital facilities that suffered the most structural damage had been built before tougher hospital construction standards had been adopted.

Shortly after the Northridge earthquake, and largely in response to it, Senator Alfred Alquist led an effort to get the California Legislature to enact legislation to enhance seismic safety in existing acute care hospitals. The resulting legislation came to be called SB 1953 (Senate Bill 1953). It created a staged implementation scheme in which acute care hospital buildings built before 1973 and classified as most susceptible to seismic damage and loss of life would be strengthened to enhance their post-earthquake functionality and safety or be taken out of service by January 1, 2008. By 2030, all acute care facilities built before 1973 were supposed to be replaced with new facilities meeting contemporary seismic safety standards. SB 1953, essentially an amendment to the 1972 Alquist Act, became law in January 1995, after being approved by the California legislature in September 1994.

The California Office of Statewide Hospital Planning and Development (OSHPD) was assigned the task of developing administrative regulations to define the program and with implementing it. The regulations intended to implement the SB 1953 were published on March 18, 1998 (OSHPD 1998), at which time OSHPD initiated its implementation efforts.

On the face of it, who could object to wanting acute care hospitals "up to speed" in terms of seismic safety? Society is not well served if these buildings collapse because of an earthquake or if they are nonfunctional following an earthquake. General expectations are that patients and staff should be safe during earthquakes, and that facilities should be open and available for treating those injured by earthquakes. If a facility is damaged by an earthquake, it can be out of service for an extended period. Hospitals that are out of service cannot fulfill their primary function of serving their community. Depending on the size of the community, a given hospital may be the only one within reasonable driving distance for a significant number of residents. This was the case when the Olive View Hospital failed during the 1971 Sylmar Earthquake.

Public policy intervention seems appropriate in this case. Healthcare facilities have been regulated for a long time, largely because of their societal importance. Give their special social importance, ensuring that hospitals are safe and can function when most needed warrants government involvement, regardless of the hospital's ownership (i.e., whether owned by non-profit, government, or investor-owned organizations). SB 1953 provided what appeared to seismic safety advocates a reasonable time line within which to address what many people might consider a serious problem in a state where moderate earthquakes occur frequently and with the likelihood of several occurring in the course of a building's normal life span.

Still, a large number of significant problems arose, resulting in delays in the implementation timetable. As we suggested earlier, few things are as simple as they seem. Or as simple as one might hope.

Quite independently of California's legislative activities, the National Science Foundation created three national centers for earthquake engineering research in the late 1980s. One of the three, the Multi-Disciplinary Center for Earthquake Engineering Research (MCEER), was headquartered at the University at Buffalo, part of the State University of New York. Although centered in Buffalo, MCEER involved faculty and researchers from across the country. MCEER, prompted in part by the extensive damage suffered by acute care hospital facilities in the January 1994 Northridge Earthquake, was particularly interested in seismic safety in hospitals. Much of the Center's work focused on engineering technology that would improve the performance of buildings subjected to earthquake forces, but MCEER was also interested in the challenges of moving technical knowledge to actual application, particularly in existing structures. An official of California's OSHPD who was serving on MCEER's external Advisory Committee suggested to MCEER managers that the implementation of the 1994 California legislation would provide an excellent opportunity to study implementation. Hence, the authors began their case study in 1999.

The timing of the research has been particularly propitious. SB 1953 provides an exceptional and timely opportunity to study a large-scale attempt to enhance seismic safety in existing buildings in real time. We have been able to track the program and the responses of hospital owners and other constituent groups as the case has developed, rather than attempting to do so retrospectively from records and individuals' recollections. Thus, we have conducted our case study from 1999 into 2011, tracking events and analyzing how various aspects of the case have emerged and fared through that time.

The SB 1953 story is still unfolding. It is expected to continue to unfold until 2030 and perhaps beyond. That year is the target year for all acute care hospitals in California to be fully compliant with contemporary structural and nonstructural seismic safety requirements. If history is a guide, we suspect that "unfinished business" will remain at the end of 2030.

The SB 1953 case is particularly informative. California has a long history of enacting and trying to implement legislation requiring retrofit of existing, privately owned buildings. Keeping those various laws and ordinances requiring retrofit in force and implementing the policies has been particularly difficult, even in California, where frequent earthquakes remind residents of their vulnerability. Moreover, extraordinary changes have occurred in the healthcare industry during administration of SB 1953. Thus, the case presents an excellent opportunity to facilitate examination of our three fundamental questions. The findings certainly have salience for hazard mitigation efforts, but, beyond that, contribute significantly to understanding public policy implementation more generally.

1.6 Our Research Approach

This research does not constitute a policy or program evaluation of SB 1953. Were it such, the focus would have been considerably different. The work began and was completed as an effort to answer the three questions posed at the beginning of the chapter. In our efforts to answer those questions, we focused much more on programmatic outcomes rather than on program administration. One of the very useful aspects of this case is that only one agency, California's Officc of Statewide Health Planning and Development (OSHPD), was responsible for administering the program. This fact held constant one of the variables thought to affect implementation – the involvement of multiple agencies at multiple levels of government. It enabled us to look at the history leading to and the development of the Act and to focus on various aspects of why things happened as they did.

We began our work with an extensive search and review of the scholarly literature on implementation of public policies (Alesch and Petak 2001). Following that review, we conducted a series of initial discussions with parties involved in creating and implementing SB 1953 and with healthcare professionals faced with complying with the law. When we assessed the results of those interviews, we concluded that we could not answer our three fundamental questions within the framework of the existing literature on public policy implementation. The literature was confined, largely, to a set of variables of mainly marginal relevance to the apparent challenges with SB 1953.

We concluded that our case study could not constitute a test of hypotheses based on extant theories of policy implementation. Thus, we decided that our research would be aimed at building grounded theory embracing additional kinds of variables. It was clear that to answer our three fundamental questions, it would be necessary to focus first on learning how the case was unfolding and why it was unfolding as it was. We decided that the best way for us to do this was to talk directly with participants in the process to see how they made sense of what had happened and what was happening from their perspectives as public policy makers, as public administrators, and as owners and managers of organizations targeted by the hazard mitigation regulations. Thus, we embarked on a quest for greater understanding of a complex set of actors, issues, processes, and choices. All have continued to evolve in a dynamic context.

Our primary method of obtaining information was from semi-structured, open-ended, and repeated rounds of interviews with key stakeholders. Following each round of interviews, we reviewed what we had heard, discussed it, reached tentative conclusions about various aspects of the case, and then, went back to the literature. We examined the literature not only on implementation, but also on organizational behavior, behavioral models of decision making, and of other case studies to learn what others have said about the phenomena we observed. We reviewed public records and statistical reports. We went back to many of those we interviewed to pursue points of clarification. We wrote draft pieces and asked participants in the process to comment on them in terms of the accuracy of facts and our interpretation of those facts.

We have attempted to capture the story of SB 1953 and to interpret why things have happened as they have, and what we might learn from the experience, particularly as it applies to developing and implementing regulatory policy intended to reduce the likely adverse consequences of hazardous events.

We count ourselves fortunate that, even as we were attempting to gain understanding into the complexities of policy implementation, others had reached conclusions similar to ours about implementation in the broader sense. Ultimately, we pursued a research agenda that reflected new thinking about a continuing concern. Essentially, that agenda is outlined in Hill and Hupe (2002, p. 7) when they call to mind Mazmanian and Sabatier stating that implementation "normally runs through a number of stages." These begin "with passage of the basic statute, followed by the policy inputs (decisions) of the implementing agencies, the compliance of target groups with those decisions, the actual impacts – both intended and unintended – of those outputs, the perceived impacts of agency decisions, and finally, important revisions (or attempted revisions) in the basic statute" (1983, pp. 20–21). Reinforced by what others were writing, we felt confident in our chosen course of action.

The SB 1953 program is not scheduled to be completed until 2030 and, as we write this, it is only 2011. It will be two more decades before all California acute care hospitals are supposed to meet contemporary seismic standards. Thus, this is actually a "mid-point" assessment. For our purposes, however, the SB 1953 experience from 1994 to 2010 seems sufficient to address our fundamental questions.

1.7 The Plan of the Book

The plan of the book is simple. The chapters immediately following this introduction comprise Part I. Part I provides essential background information on California's attempts to cause other governments and private actors within the State to upgrade buildings built before seismic safety codes were strengthened. It describes the activities and events leading up to the enactment of SB 1953 and what happened during more than a decade following enactment, and where things stood at the end of 2010, 16 years after enactment in 1994.

Part II focuses on our conclusions about three sets of factors that affect policy implementation, particularly as it relates to hazard mitigation. First, we look at the actions of the agency or agencies charged with policy and program administration. Second, we examine the response of the regulated organizations – in this case health-care organizations – and on our understanding of how organizations make hazard mitigation investment decisions. Finally, we look at what we choose to call problem definition and policy design and the implications for that in a dynamic context.

Part V consists of a single chapter in which we describe what we call the "ecology of public policy implementation."

References

Alesch DJ, Petak WJ (2001) Overcoming obstacles to implementing earthquake hazard mitigation policies: stage 1 report. Technical report MCEER-01-0004. Multidisciplinary Center for Earthquake Engineering Research, Buffalo

Bardach E (1977) The implementation game: what happens after a bill becomes law. The MIT Press, Cambridge

Berman P (1980) Thinking about programmed and adaptive implementation: matching strategies to situations. In: Ingram HM, Mann DE (eds) Why policies succeed or fail. Sage, Beverley Hills

Burby RJ, May PJ, Paterson RC (1998) Improving compliance with regulations: choices and outcomes for local government. APA J 64(3):324–334

Calista D (1994) Policy implementation. In: Nagel S (ed) Encyclopedia of policy studies. Marcel Dekker, New York, pp 117–155

Greil A (2010) Disasters in 2010 costs insurance industry $36 billion. Wall Str J (citing Swiss Re), 30 Nov 2010

Gunderson LH, Holling CS (eds) (2002) Panarchy: understanding transformations in human and natural systems. Island Press, Washington, DC

Hill HC (2003) Understanding implementation: street-level bureaucrats' resources for reform. J Public Adm Theory 13(3):265–282

Hill M, Hupe P (2002) Implementing public policy: governance in theory and in practice. Sage Publications, Thousand Oaks

Lipsky M (1971) Street level bureaucracy and the analysis of urban reform. Urban Aff Quart 6:391–409

Majone G, Wildavsky A (1978) Implementation as evolution. In: Policy studies review, 1978 ed. Sage Publications, Beverly Hills, pp 109–114

Mazmanian DA, Sabatier PA (1989) Implementation of public policy. University of America Press, New York

Office of Technology Assessment, US Congress (1995) Reducing earthquake losses, OTA-ETI-623. US Government Printing Office, Washington, DC, Sept 1995

OSHPD (1998) Seismic retrofit program – SB1953. State of California, Office of Statewide Healthcare Planning, Sacramento. Retrieved 2 June 2005 from http://www.oshpd.ca.gov/fdd/sb1953/index.htm

Pfeffer J, Sutton RI (2000) The knowing-doing gap: how smart companies turn knowledge into action. Harvard Business School Press, Cambridge

Pressman JL, Wildavski AB (1973) Implementation: how great expectations in Washington are dashed in Oakland. University of California Press: Berkely, CA

Rein M, Rabinowitz FF (1978) Implementation: a theoretical perspective. In: Burnham WD, Weinberg MW (eds) American politics and public policy. MIT Press, Cambridge

Schultz CH, Koenig KL, Lewis RJ (2003) Implications of hospital evacuation after the Northridge, California, earthquake. N Engl J Med 348:1349–1355

Part I
SB 1953: The Origins and the Experience Through 2010

Part I describes the history leading to enactment of SB 1953, California's amendment to and furtherance of the Alfred E. Alquist Hospital Seismic Safety Act of 1983 and tracks program implementation from 1998 through 2010. How this natural hazards mitigation policy came into being and the implementation experience over its first 12 years provides the basis for the balance of the book in which the authors explore the primary obstacles to program implementation and means for overcoming those obstacles.

Chapter 2
Origins and History of California Seismic Building Retrofit Regulations

2.1 In the Beginning

California has a long history of enacting legislation to regulate how local governments and private organizations constructed buildings to enhance their resistance to earthquakes. This was most often done at the behest of science and engineering advocates and in direct response to earthquake events. California's history of enacting legislation to force building owners to retrofit or replace buildings constructed before those regulations were put into place is also long but has followed a more difficult, perhaps more tortuous path. The history of the State's efforts provides insights into the origins and the continuing story of SB 1953.

The first seismic building code in the United States was enacted December 17, 1925 by the Santa Barbara City Council just 6 months after the Santa Barbara Earthquake of June, 1925. Not long after, in April 1926, 20 years after the Great San Francisco Earthquake of 1906, the City of Palo Alto, California, followed suit by adopting an amendment to its building code requiring earthquake resistant construction. These codes formalized seismic design practice at the time. The 1925 earthquake in Santa Barbara brought focus to the problem of building construction in earthquake country and led to the adoption of the new codes by these two communities. It also helped keep the matter of seismic safety alive in the years following the 1906 earthquake, especially through the activism of a few people in the scientific and engineering community.

Following the San Francisco earthquake, civic boosters and promoters convinced many that the real problem had been the fire that followed the earthquake and not the earthquake itself. Others, building on the lack of significant knowledge of seismology and in collaboration with the Building Owners and Managers Association, were able to convince the City of Los Angeles Chamber of Commerce and others that there had been an overreaction to the earthquake threat. With support from the Building Owners and Managers Association, a 1928 book, *Southern California Geology and Los Angeles Earthquakes*, was authored by a petroleum geologist.

D.J. Alesch et al., *Natural Hazard Mitigation Policy: Implementation, Organizational Choice, and Contextual Dynamics*, Environmental Hazards,
DOI 10.1007/978-94-007-2235-4_2,

This book frustrated the efforts of seismic safety advocates and led to the belief that the Southern California area was "not-only free from a probability of severe seismic disturbances, but has the least to fear from 'Acts of God' of any city under the American flag" (Geschwind 2001, pp. 79–94).

Early in the morning 1 day in 1933, Long Beach experienced an earthquake which was later estimated to be magnitude 6.2 on the Richter scale. That earthquake helped to overcome the belief that California was safe from earthquakes and reactivated concern for seismic safety. The earthquake caused 120 deaths and extensive property damage (about $400 million in 2001 dollars) (Geschwind 2001). Further, the temblor destroyed 70 schools and damaged 120 other school buildings, of which 41 were rendered unsafe for occupancy and were closed permanently. Since school was not in session when the early morning earthquake occurred, no children were injured while attending school. However, the possibility of many casualties among school children caused great concern. That concern manifested itself in the California legislature adopting the Field Act, which gave the State the power to approve public school construction plans, inspect ongoing construction, and inspect existing school buildings.

2.1.1 The Field Act of 1933

C. Don Field, a California assemblyman from Los Angeles County, proposed draft legislation on March 22, 1933 that was adopted shortly thereafter on April 10, 1933. The impetus for what became known as the Field Act was from "parents outraged over the widespread collapse of school buildings during the Long Beach earthquake" (Geschwind 2001, p. 113). The Field Act (California Education Code Sections 39140, et seq.) was intended to assure that all public schools in the State were safe in earthquakes. It established minimum seismic design criteria for schools, required that structural design of school buildings be done by structural engineers knowledgeable in earthquake engineering, and called for strict checking of plans by the State with thorough inspection of construction.

In many ways, the Field Act was patterned after the State's Dam Safety Act (California Water Code, Sections 6000-6501), which was passed after the 1928 collapse of the St. Francis Dam that caused extensive property damage and 420 deaths. Most notable about that legislation was the shift from local government oversight to State oversight of all non-federal dams. In brief, the State assumed responsibility for reviewing all dam design and construction elements in order to ensure safety. With respect to the Field Act, all new schools were subject to the new controls, but, importantly, there were no provisions to force reinforcement or replacement of the existing inventory of schools throughout the State, many of which were built of unreinforced masonry. This new Act became the "major government bulwark for the establishment of seismic safety in California" (Geschwind 2001, p. 114).

2.1.2 *Riley Act of 1933*

In addition to concern about schools, concern existed about the safety of other kinds of buildings in California. This concern led the Structural Engineers Association of Northern California to draft a bill, a modified version of the Field Act, to require all buildings in the State to incorporate seismic resistant construction. The legislation that followed came to be known as the Riley Act of 1933. It was essentially submitted to the California Legislature as early as March 1933 (Geschwind 2001, p. 114). Assemblyman Riley of Long Beach submitted a revised version to the legislature on April 25, 1933, which was adopted May 27, 1933. The Riley Act was supported by structural engineers and architects across California and by State Chambers of Commerce.

However, as early as 1935 there were attempts by elected officials and business interests to weaken both the Field and Riley Acts because, they maintained, earthquake hazards were exaggerated and the legislation created personal liability concerns among school board members (Geschwind 2001, p. 117). Further, since "enforcement of the act was left to local building inspection departments, which were generally understaffed, the Act was often left unenforced" (Geschwind 2001, p. 114). Despite these issues, the Riley Act was credited with compelling "official acknowledgement that earthquakes do happen in California" (Geschwind 2001, p. 114).

2.1.3 *Garrison Act of 1939*

The Garrison Act was an attempt to address the hazardous conditions that existed following the Field Act because that Act did not address seismic safety in schools built before adoption of the Act. The Garrison Act required that seismic evaluations on all school buildings built before 1933 be completed by 1970. Those buildings were to be retrofitted to meet Field Act standards or abandoned by June 30, 1975. Due to limited resources and the absence of an effective enforcement mechanism, there was, in fact, only limited progress toward accomplishing the stated goal of removing hazardous buildings from the inventory of facilities used for schools.

The Garrison Act removed personal liability for damage or injury caused by an earthquake from school board members if their good faith efforts to raise funds for strengthening existing schools were defeated in school bond referenda. In essence, Geschwind (2001, p. 117) argues, it "removed the incentive driving strengthening of existing schools." Advocates and individuals in the Office of State Division of Architecture were vigilant in maintaining core provisions of the Field and Garrison Acts. Nonetheless, in 1963, the legislature quietly removed the waiver of liability from school board members (via the California Government Tort Claims Act of 1963). Most school boards avoided the whole issue, including the issue of liability, by not ordering school inspections and by constructing new schools to meet the demand of baby boomers.

In 1966, however, California's Attorney General ruled that failure to request a structural inspection constituted negligence and exposed school board members to personal liability. School boards again started to pressure the legislature for relief from liability (Geschwind 2001, p. 186). The 1967 legislature obliged, via Assembly Bill 450 (sponsored by Assemblyman Leroy Greene), and re-instituted the waiver of liability originally provided by the Garrison Act (Geschwind 2001, p. 186). The waiver applied, however, only if school boards required inspection of all old building by 1970 and sought bond or tax increases to finance retrofit at least once every 5 years until approved (Geschwind 2001, p. 186).

2.1.4 The Greene Act of 1968

The Greene Act of 1968 (Assembly Bill 420) required California school districts to comply with the Garrison Act of 1939 (Geschwind 2001, p. 186). School buildings not retrofitted or meeting Field Act standards were to be abandoned by 1975. This put pressure on school boards to find money. If they failed to find money to retrofit or rebuild the facilities, they had to put students into temporary buildings or in double sessions in adequate buildings once the 1975 deadline passed.

2.2 Pre-existing Buildings and Other Complexities

In the mid-1960s, California State officials estimated that between 15% and 20% of old, pre-1933 schools in the school building inventory needed seismic retrofit (Geschwind 2001, pp. 186–189). In 1966, the estimated cost to retrofit those old school buildings was estimated as low as $1.2 billion and as high as $3 billion. Many architects, engineers, contractors, and labor unions endorsed efforts to raise money, but, then, in addition to concerns about the safety of children and school staff, they stood to gain from retrofitting. Legislation compelling retrofits of existing buildings was likely to be perceived, at least by some, as a "full employment act" for these professionals.

The California Property Tax Revolt of the 1960s was another obstacle to replacing or strengthening the old schools still in the inventory. The revolt was a political movement aimed at limiting property tax increases. It resulted in State legislation limiting increases in property taxes by limiting the rate at which governments could increase the assessed valuation of property that remained in the hands of an owner. The assessment on property that changed hands or that was newly created was adjusted to reflect the purchase price, but was subsequently subject to the limited increase provisions. Property tax revenue did not increase in proportion to government costs. Voters rejected referenda calling for borrowing or tax increases to provide money for retrofitting. The job of raising the necessary money was made even tougher with a 1971 State Supreme Court ruling that affirmed that a two-thirds majority vote set forth in the California constitution was required for local bond issues to pass. In 1972, State Senator George Moscone introduced a bill for a state referendum (Proposition 9, November 7, 1972) to reduce the required vote to a simple majority for money to retrofit schools. The proposition won 54.5% of the votes, and passed (Geschwind 2001, p. 189). The change increased the success rate for bond measures and accelerated retrofitting. However, 1,593 pre-Field Act buildings were still being used in California in 1972 (Geschwind 2001, p. 189). Tax protesters argued that the concern about seismic effects on school buildings was a ploy by schools to get money for other purposes, not for retrofit. In fact, many school districts did add money to proposed referenda to include other measures to bring schools up to more modern educational standards.

In 1974, the California legislature passed Assembly Bill 2615 (sponsored again by Assemblyman Greene), which extended the deadline to 1977 for replacing school buildings that did not comply with Field Act standards for districts with extenuating circumstances. By 1977, only 19 school buildings located in rural areas remained to be retrofitted (Geschwind 2001, p. 189). The process of removing unsafe schools from the California inventory required extraordinary efforts by seismic safety advocates for half a century. They needed State mandated retrofitting, State changes in the rules for bond issues, and, ultimately, State funding.

2.3 Threats to the Field Act Program and Primary Barriers to Success

Historically, according to Dennis Bellet, Chief Structural Engineer, California Division of the State Architect, two principal barriers limited the success of the Field Act. "First, funding for school construction is unstable and the quantity of work often exceeds staff capacity and schedule pressures can lead to less aggressive inspection and less rigorous plan review. Second, the 1933 Field Act does not adequately address the risk posed by nonstructural elements, which often come loose and fall during moderate earthquakes" (Bellet 2004, p. 153).

Attempts continue today to adopt legislation to remove the requirements of the Field Act for certain types of buildings (e.g., California community colleges), in part because at least some stakeholders believe that "aggressive plan review and construction inspection is too costly or time consuming" (Bellet 2004, p. 153). Specifically, because of what was perceived as the limited requirements of the Uniform Building Code (UBC) and the variability of the code's enforcement by local governments, the Field Act requires that the design and construction of K-12 school and community college buildings be regulated by the California State Architect rather than local government building departments. In general, buildings constructed to the UBC standards are designed to withstand an earthquake in order to allow the occupants to exit safely. Buildings constructed to Field Act standards are designed to withstand an earthquake in order to allow the occupants to exit safely *and* for the building to remain usable.

The differences in building construction standards between the Field Act and the UBC have diminished because of increases in the requirements of the UBC. There are, however, significant differences in the enforcement of the standards (Seismic Safety Commission 2004). "Under the Field Act, a qualified professional licensed in California (i.e., structural engineers at the Division of the State Architect (DSA)) must review and approve construction plans. The Field Act also requires, during the construction phase of a project, that a DSA-certified inspector continuously inspect the project to ensure compliance with the plans and structural safety standards" (California State Assembly Hearing Record 2004). Enforcement is by the on-site Inspector-of-Record (certified by the DSA, yet retained and accountable to the local school district), while the UBC is enforced solely by the local government's building code department. A 1992 DSA study estimated that the requirements of the Field Act increase total project costs by less than 4% (Bellet 2004), and most of the difference in cost is seen as a function of increased design review time and associated construction time.

Nonetheless, the California Community Colleges have continued to argue that it is too expensive for them to build facilities in compliance with the Field Act. A number of bills have been introduced over the past several years to the State Legislature to address the concerns of the Community Colleges. Arguments in support of the various bills are best summarized by State Senator Denham, the author of Senate Bill 1175 (2004), who stated,

> Community College Boards need the flexibility to cut costs outside the classroom. This legislation allows districts to choose whether they will build facilities to the standards required of K-12 schools (Field Act) or the University of California and California State University (California Building Standards Code – CBC) (California State Assembly Hearing Record 2004).

Likewise, arguments in opposition have been expressed by the California Seismic Safety Commission.

> The Commission believes that the Field Act is critical to preserving the safety of students, faculty and staff that use school facilities every day. . . California's experience with earthquakes indisputably demonstrates that buildings constructed in accordance with the Field Act have *superior* performance during and after earthquakes (California State Assembly Hearing Record 2004) (emphasis added by the authors).

Table 2.1 summarizes the most recent bills and their disposition. A review of the issues associated with implementing post-earthquake legislation to retrofit and replace unreinforced masonry school buildings in California demonstrates the historical difficulty with implementing earthquake mitigation legislation in California, even when it is supported strongly by advocates and other stakeholders (in the case of schools, parents). This historical perspective helps to provide an understanding of the political and socio-economic issues involved with implementing past post-earthquake legislation requiring retrofit and replacement of certain types of buildings, and provides insight into the issues that influenced the implementation SB 1953. A basic question that remains unanswered is whether society has learned from experience or whether it is faced with traveling, yet again, the troubled road to

Table 2.1 Summary of recent legislative actions to remove California community colleges from the requirements of the Field Act

Bill	Disposition
SB 1175 (2004)	Authorize certain school buildings constructed after 1/1/05 on a community college campus and designed by the community college district as buildings that potentially will be used to house classes of California State University (CSU) or the University of California (UC) in addition to housing community college classes, to be built according to the provisions of the Field Act or the California Building Standards Commission's California Building Standards Code (CBSC). Passed in Senate, but not in Assembly.
AB 3010 (2004)	The Assembly Higher Education Committee passed AB 3010 on April 20, 2004, on a 7-0 vote. Required the State Architect to review plans for community college facilities at the design stage. Would have given the State Architect responsibility for engaging the designers of community college buildings in the design process, rather than only at the end of design. Overall costs expected to be lower because early plan review should catch needed plan changes earlier in the design process when they are easier and less costly to correct. However, buildings must still be built in accordance with the greater protections of the Field Act. Vetoed by the Governor on September 18, 2004.
SB 242 (2003)	Would have allowed a community college building to be built in accordance with either the Field Act or the Uniform Building Code, if the building is used to house classes offered by a community college and either the UC or the CSU, and if the building is constructed after January 1, 2004. Vetoed by the Governor citing support for the Field Act.
AB 484 (2002)	Authorized community college facilities designed for joint-use with the CSU or the UC, to be built in accordance with either the Field Act or the CBSC. Vetoed by the Governor citing support for the Field Act.
AB 2007 (2000)	Would have exempted a specific joint-use facility at Antelope Valley College from the provisions of the Field Act. Vetoed by the Governor citing support for the Field Act.
AB 80 (1999)	Would have exempted the construction and renovation of community college facilities from the requirements of the Field Act and instead required these facilities to conform to the UBC. AB 80 passed the Assembly but the author chose not to have it heard in the Senate.

Source: California Legislature, Web Site of Bill Information

devising and implementing program after program to remove critical, yet presumably unsafe, buildings from the inventory. This case study of SB 1953 is intended to take interested stakeholders closer to answering this question.

References

Bellet D (2004) Chapter 10. In: Proceedings of the Ad Hoc experts' group meeting on earthquake safety in schools, OECD Programme on educational buildings and geohazards international, OECD, Paris, 9–11 Feb. http://www.oecd.org/dataoecd/44/19/33629183.pdf

California Education Code, State of California Statutes, Sections 39140, et seq.

California State Assembly Hearing Record (2004) State of California, Sacramento

California Water Code, State of California Statutes, Sections 6000–6501

Geschwind C (2001) California earthquakes: science, risk and the politics of hazard mitigation. The John Hopkins University Press, Baltimore

Seismic Safety Commission (2004) Seismic safety in California's schools: findings and recommendations on seismic safety policies and requirements for public, private, and charter schools. State of California, Sacramento, December

State of California, Legislature Web Site of Bill Information. SB 1175 (2004), AB 3010 (2004), SB 242 (2003), AB 484 (2002), AB 2007 (2000), AB 80 (1999) (http://www.leginfo.ca.gov/bilinfo.html)

Chapter 3
The Road to SB 1953

Just as the 1933 Field Act established standards for building new schools but ignored school buildings that were built before that date, the Alquist Hospital Facilities Seismic Safety Act of 1973 established standards for building new acute care hospitals but ignored hospital buildings that were built before it was enacted. Hospitals build before 1973 were not required to meet the seismic safety standards adopted for hospitals built subsequent to that year. And, just as in the case of school buildings, decades later, many acute care hospitals built before 1973 were still in use for their original purpose. And, just as with the case of schools built before new, more rigorous standards were enacted, efforts began to remove those old acute care hospitals from use.

The law that came to be known as SB 1953 did not arise in a vacuum. Its origins lie deep within Californians' concerns about earthquake safety and it emerged from a long series of events. The chain of events leading to SB 1953 is described in this chapter.

3.1 Waypoints Along the Road to Enactment

3.1.1 Waypoint 1. Formation of the Joint Committee on Seismic Safety

The difficulties experienced in achieving legislative goals of the Field and Garrison Acts led, ultimately, to the establishment of the Joint Committee on Seismic Safety on August 25, 1969 (Senate Concurrent Resolution 128, State of California Senate 1969). The creation of the California Legislature's Joint Committee on Seismic Safety (JCSS) was an important event because it set the stage for direct input into the legislative process on issues of hospital safety by professional stakeholders, including structural engineers who became active advocates for hospital seismic safety.

D.J. Alesch et al., *Natural Hazard Mitigation Policy: Implementation, Organizational Choice, and Contextual Dynamics*, Environmental Hazards,
DOI 10.1007/978-94-007-2235-4_3, © Springer Science+Business Media B.V. 2012

The Joint Committee was directed to prepare a detailed report on seismic safety in California to be completed no later than June 30, 1974. The Resolution creating the Joint Committee called for establishing several advisory groups to assist in preparing the report for submission from the JCSS to the Legislature. The combined advisory groups were chaired by Karl V. Steinbrugge, a noted civil and structural engineer and Professor of Structural Design at the University of California at Berkeley until his retirement in 1978. At the time of his appointment as chair of the committee, Steinbrugge was president of the Earthquake Engineering Research Institute (1968–1970). He would later serve as the first chairman of the California State Seismic Safety Commission (1975–1980). The individual advisory groups and their chairs were as follows:

- **Advisory Group on Engineering Considerations and Earthquake Sciences.** This group of 14 members was directed to review available scientific and engineering knowledge relative to the reduction of the risks and damage due to earthquake and related geologic hazards. Gordon B. Oakeshott, Chair.
- **Advisory Group on Disaster Preparedness.** This 17 member group was responsible for reviewing the adequacy of existing disaster plans as far as they related to earthquakes. Robert A. Olson, Chair.
- **Advisory Group on Post-Earthquake Recovery and Redevelopment.** This group of 15 members was responsible for recommending general contingency plans to guide the long-term work of recovery, reconstruction, and redevelopment following an earthquake. Will H. Perry, Jr., Chair.
- **Advisory Group on Land Use Planning.** This group of 15 members was to determine limitations that should be placed on land development in seismically active areas and restrictions appropriate for inclusion into city, county and state governed land use plans. George G. Mader, Chair.
- **Advisory Group on Government Organization and Performance.** This group of 15 members was charged with assessing how various governmental organizations were to be involved in implementing the plans formulated by the advisory groups. Marcella Jacobson, Chair.

3.1.2 Waypoint 2. The February 9, 1971 San Fernando (Sylmar) Earthquake

The Sylmar earthquake (magnitude 6.6) was a significant temblor. It jolted not only residents, but policy makers as well. The San Fernando Veterans Administration Hospital, built of unreinforced masonry in 1925 and never retrofitted, collapsed during the earthquake with the loss of 49 lives. Other hospitals experienced significant damage as well.

The Olive View Hospital in the San Fernando Valley was virtually brand new, having been dedicated just a month before the earthquake. Nonetheless, substantial structural and nonstructural damage occurred. Three exterior stairwells and a portico structure over the ambulance parking area collapsed. The collapsing portico killed one person. The first floor design did not have sufficient strength or toughness to withstand lateral forces caused by the earthquake. The main structure design involved a "soft story" first floor architectural design, consisting of a large open space frame. The building suffered significant damage and required total replacement. Holy Cross Hospital and Pacoima Memorial Lutheran Hospital were also seriously damaged. The damage to hospitals and the number of lives lost in the Veterans Administration Hospital raised concerns over future potential loss of life, treatment facilities, and capacity to meet healthcare needs following a subsequent earthquake. Steinbrugge and his colleagues, writing the report for the Pacific Fire Rating Bureau on the San Fernando Earthquake, stated:

> Surely public interest is much better served if hospital structures are designed with sufficient damage control features so as to remain functional after an event. This means not only placing severe limits on permissible structural damage, but also severe limits on permissible elevator damage, telephone and other communications damage, standby power damage and the like (Steinbrugge et al. 1971: 56).

This statement by Steinbrugge and his colleagues in 1971 was essentially the problem statement underlying the legislation enacted in 1973 and in SB 1953 enacted more than 20 years later. The wording of the problem statement, as we will see in a subsequent chapter, remained essentially the same, almost word for word.

On August 27, 1971, the Joint Rules Committee of the California Legislature adopted Resolution Seven, charging the Joint Committee on Seismic Safety with establishing a Special Sub-Committee to study the San Fernando Earthquake of February 9, 1971. The resolution allocated $150,000 from the contingent funds of the Senate and Assembly to be used in the investigation. This Special Sub-Committee called upon the Advisory Groups of the JCSS to assist by providing technical information on the San Fernando Earthquake, including suggestions for legislation that could mitigate the damage caused by a similar earthquake in the future. The Sub-Committee provided the Legislature with a preliminary report on July 31, 1971 and a final report in December 1972.

The Joint Committee's detailed report on seismic safety in California, *Meeting the Earthquake Challenge: The Final Report to the Legislature*, due at the end of 1972, was actually completed in January of 1974 (State of California, Joint Commission on Seismic Safety 1974). The major emphasis of the Joint Committee on Seismic Safety's work shifted at that time to drafting and proposing legislation based on the suggestions made in the Joint Committee's report on how to mitigate California's earthquake risks. The shift in focus led to the development of groups of technical professionals concerned with reducing earthquake risk through improved building standards and codes. Twenty-three *ad hoc* groups were formed to facilitate the legislative drafting and lobbying process. The groups drew their membership largely from the JCSS's Advisory Groups. The groups operated essentially autonomously, but were called on to report to the Joint Committee on Seismic Safety.

3.1.3 Waypoint 3. The Hospital Facilities Seismic Safety Act of 1973 (Senate Bill 519)

The Hospital Facilities Seismic Safety Act of 1973 Act was not enacted in the immediate aftermath of the February 1971 San Fernando earthquake. Geschwind concludes that experience shows that the evolution of hazard mitigation is not a simple story of immediate response to natural disasters, but "new measures trickled out over a course of years" (Geschwind 2001, p. 228). Also important is the "degree to which mitigation advocates have been organized and have had the resources necessary to mobilize public opinion or the political process in pursuit of their goals" (Geschwind 2001, p. 229).

Initial impetus for the Hospital Facilities Seismic Safety Act of 1973 came from J. Meehan, the chief structural engineer for the Schoolhouse Section, State Office of Architecture and Construction, which was responsible for enforcing the Field Act. Meehan proposed to the Joint Committee in January 1971 that the Field Act provisions be extended to hospitals. Senator Alfred Alquist moved to introduce a bill incorporating Meehan's suggestions (Geschwind 2001, p. 176).

The California State Department of Public Health objected to the bill because it already had power to approve and supervise hospital construction and did not want to cede control over structural matters to the Schoolhouse Section of the State Office of Architecture and Construction. The agency argued that doing so would fragment the process of approving hospital plans. Alquist consulted with the Joint Committee where engineers argued that public health officials did not have sufficient expertise in structural engineering enabling them to enforce seismic design requirements. Finally, Alquist amended his bill to provide Public Health with ultimate plan approval but required Public Health to subcontract to the Schoolhouse Section of State Office of Architecture for seismic review (Geschwind 2001, p. 176).

Public Health objected to that provision and, with help from the California Hospital Association (and the City of San Francisco which argued it would cost too much), got the Senate Finance Committee to kill the bill. Alquist reintroduced the bill in the 1972 legislative session, amended to meet the Public Health Department's objection by creating a Hospital Building Safety Board under the control of the Public Health Department's director and with a hospital administrator as a member of the Board. These changes led to passage and adoption. In approving the Hospital Facilities Seismic Safety Act (HFSSA), the Legislature noted that,

> Hospitals that house patients who have less than the capacity of normally healthy persons to protect themselves, and that must be reasonably capable of providing services to the public after a disaster, shall be designed and constructed to *resist, insofar as practical, the forces generated by earthquakes*, gravity and winds (State of California, California Statutes 1973) (emphasis added by authors).

This statement echoes the problem statement posed by Steinbrugge and his colleagues in the report they issued in 1971. The wording is paraphrased, but the sense that hospitals must be reasonably capable of functioning in their intended roles following an earthquake is reinforced. At the same time, the statement simply refers to the need for the buildings to withstand the forces of earthquakes, wind, and gravity, without any indication of the levels of shaking and wind against which the buildings ought to be expected to continue to function.

It took two legislative attempts for the HFSSA to be adopted. A major issue was the initial call for "immediate strengthening or replacement of all health care facilities that did not meet modern standards" (Poland 1994, p. 114). Recognizing the economic difficulty associated with retrofitting all health care facilities, the bill was changed to require retrofit of only those facilities that were to undergo significant remodeling. Following the experience gained from the Field Act, it was decided that the best approach would be to require a single set of statewide standards to be administered by the State rather than have local officials responsible for such structures within their jurisdictions.

The establishment of a common code and administrative process was intended to eliminate jurisdictional differences in codes and their enforcement. Independent plan checking and construction inspection processes were established as key elements in quality control (Lagorio et al. 1995, p. 7). The Hospital Facilities Seismic Safety Act (HFSSA) was to be administered by the Office of the State Architect, Office of the State Fire Marshall, and the Office of Statewide Health Planning and Development (OSHPD). Included in the HFSSA was a significant, new, and explicit policy goal: that hospitals were to be designed such that they would control damage and "remain functional following an earthquake." This overall goal led to concern by professional engineers that "damage control" would be interpreted as "earthquake proof," which led to the insertion of the words "insofar as practical" to remain functional, but no one at that time attempted to operationalize what "insofar as practical" actually meant.

Based largely on the experience with the Field Act and J. Meehan's influence, the 1973 Hospital Facilities Seismic Safety Act was generally patterned after the Field Act. It specified that the State Division of Architecture would be responsible for implementation (i.e., the same State review agency as for schools), and further stipulated that buildings were to be designed by structural engineers registered in California. The HFSSA included four main components:

1. Geologic hazard studies for sites,
2. Use of structural design standards against forces in excess of those used for "normal" buildings,
3. Specific design requirements for nonstructural elements, and,
4. Strict review of design and inspection of construction.

In order to address concerns by the Office of Health Planning and Development (OSHPD), the Hospital Facilities Seismic Safety Act established a Hospital Building Safety Board for the purpose of advising "the Director of OSHPD on the administration of the Hospital Facilities Seismic Safety Act, and acting as a board of appeals with regard to seismic safety and fire and life safety issues relating to hospital facilities, particularly in matters relating to the administration and enforcement of building standards relating to hospitals during construction or alteration of projects submitted to OSHPD" (State of California and Hospital Safety Building 2003).

The Board's 13 members are appointed by the Director of OSHPD from nominations submitted by professional associations, as specified in the Health and Safety Code, with three more individuals appointed as public members. Six statutory *ex officio* members representing state agencies with programs that interface with the hospital design and construction program also sit on the Board. The Director has the authority to appoint three additional *ex officio* members as desired. Board members are expected to maintain close contact with professional groups and important industry organizations in order to bring attention to changes and emerging issues occurring in the design and construction of health facilities in California.

3.1.4 Waypoint 4. Seismic Safety Commission Established in May 1975

The Joint Committee on Seismic Safety (JCSS) was officially terminated on December 31, 1974, as provided for in the 1969 Joint Resolution creating it. In its final report, the JCSS made what it said was its most significant recommendation. It proposed creation of a watchdog commission on seismic safety. It proposed that the role of such a commission would be "to develop seismic safety goals and programs, help evaluate and integrate the work of state and local agencies concerned with earthquake safety, and see that the programs are carried out effectively and the objectives are accomplished."

On February 14, 1974, State Senator Alquist introduced legislation to establish such a commission based on a draft written by Steinbrugge. Much compromise was required for enactment, as the bill proposed a strong commission. Its members would be appointed by the governor, but it would act independently. It would have the power to review state agency budgets for seismic attention, develop criteria and standards for hazard mitigation, require all agencies to comply with the standards, and it would transfer all boards established earlier (e.g., the Hospital Building Safety Board) to the Commission.

Not surprisingly, other state agencies objected strongly. Engineering associations also objected because of concern for infringement on the code writing process. Senator Alquist amended the proposed legislation to allow the Hospital Building Safety Board to remain separate and to change the Commission from a rule-making to an advisory body. Subsequently, the bill was adopted in September 1974 and the California Seismic Safety Commission was formally inaugurated in May 1975 with the swearing in of 12 members (California Codes, Government Code (1974).

3.1.5 Waypoint 5. The Palmdale Bulge

In 1976, the U.S. Geological Service (USGS) developed data suggesting that a bulge or uplift had occurred along the San Andreas Fault. Caltech scientist, James

Whitcomb, predicted that the bulge was a precursor to an earthquake in that location. Consequently, a first act of the California Seismic Safety Commission (SSC) was to recommend a survey to evaluate the anticipated seismic performance of hospitals in six counties of Southern California located near the Palmdale Bulge.

The SSC requested that the California Office of Statewide Health Planning and Development (OSHPD) survey hospital buildings in the region to ascertain the survivability of the hospital building stock should a major earthquake occur. OSHPD completed its inventory of the five-county Los Angeles area in 1982 under contract with the Office of the State Architect. The inventory consisted of a "walk-through" of hospitals and a review of available drawings. The inventory (coupled with work being done by the USGS on the Palmdale Bulge, e.g., Castle et al. 1974, 1976; Real and Bennett 1976) indicated that many hospital buildings might not be capable of continuing operations following a major earthquake.

3.1.6 Waypoint 6. The Alfred E. Alquist Hospital Facilities Seismic Safety Act of 1983

Senator Alquist, continuing his active involvement in seismic safety issues, authored legislation in 1983 to amend the 1973 Hospital Facilities Seismic Safety Act. The amendments were intended to solve some problems that had become apparent as agencies worked to administer the requirements set forth in the 1973 Act. Specifically, the amendments preempted local government building inspections for enforcing building standards published in the California Building Standards Code relating to the regulation of hospital projects. This was intended to end double inspections and fee charges as well as to eliminate conflicts between jurisdictions due to varying and conflicting interpretations of the building code. The amendments were also intended to strengthen administrative procedures and to help facilitate fund management, personnel management, and contracting.

As described by OSHPD,

> In 1983, the HSSA (Health and Safety Code, Section 129675) was significantly amended and ultimately preempted local building departments from all hospital construction plan review responsibility and transferred it the Office of Statewide Health Planning and Development (OSHPD), and the Division of the State Architect. This essentially created a building department within the Office of Statewide Health Planning, called Facilities Development Division (FDD) (Office of Statewide Health Planning and Development 2010).

The amendments designated OSHPD as "responsible for establishing, maintaining, and operating separate, but coordinated, plan review and field inspection units within the statewide office." Finally, the amendments authorized OSHPD, "with the advice of the Building Safety Board, to enter into contracts for research regarding the reduction or elimination of seismic or other safety hazards in hospital buildings or research regarding hospital building standards".

Complaints about costs associated with plan review and approval delays, complicated regulations, extensive inspections, and other factors declined during the 5-year period following the 1983 Amendments to the 1973 Act. Still, as we will see, similar complaints would accompany future legislation.

3.1.7 Waypoint 7. The California Earthquake Hazards Reduction Act of 1986 and *California at Risk*

The timing of the California Earthquake Hazards Reduction (CEHR) Act of 1986 may suggest that it was in response to the disastrous earthquake in Mexico City on September 19, 1985. Actually, work began on the bill, SB 548, and its language in February 1985. The CEHR Act required the Seismic Safety Commission (SSC) to develop a series of 5-year programs designed to significantly reduce statewide earthquake hazards by the end of the twentieth century. Conveying urgency, the law required completion of the first 5 year plan before the end of 1986, the same year it was enacted. The first 5-year program is outlined in Seismic Safety Commission's report, *California at Risk: Reducing Earthquake Hazards 1987 to 1992* (Seismic Safety Commission 1986).

California at Risk included the first formal statement about the threat posed by the continued use of hospitals built before the Hospital Facilities Seismic Safety Act of 1973 imposed new and more stringent construction standards for hospital buildings. At the time the 1973 Alquist legislation was enacted, it was expected that pre-1973 hospital buildings would be gradually withdrawn from use; however, as it turned out, they were being withdrawn at a very slow rate. It was becoming clear to seismic safety advocates that many would continue functioning as acute care hospital buildings for some time to come, barring a major earthquake. Thus, *California at Risk* addressed the problems associated with older, nonconforming hospital buildings. *California at Risk*, Initiative 1.2, states the following:

> Operators of hospitals constructed prior to the effective date for the Hospital Facilities Seismic Safety Act, regardless of ownership, should be required to strengthen and improve their ability to function following earthquake in accordance with a plan developed by the Office of Statewide Health Planning and Development (OSHPD). In undertaking these measures, OSHPD should work with organizations such as the California Hospital Association, the College of Emergency Physicians, and the Hospital Councils of Northern and Southern California to promote the concepts of functionality of hospitals following a damaging earthquake (Seismic Safety Commission 1986).

And, then,

> Hospitals must be able to function following an earthquake to provide emergency medical care. Hospital damage poses a special threat to public safety because of the high occupancy and special needs of many patients. Investments in reducing structural and nonstructural hazards are justifiable in view of the very large investments in equipment and inventory that could be irreparably damaged in a strong earthquake. The present law governing hospital seismic safety, enacted following the 1971 San Fernando earthquake, did not apply to facilities already in existence. Earthquake damage reports developed by the U.S. Geological Survey estimate that substantial losses of function would occur for hospitals in Los Angeles and Orange counties (up to one third) and the San Francisco Area (up to one half). In view

of the public's expectation that health care facilities be accessible at all times, especially after an earthquake, this program is needed (Seismic Safety Commission 1986).

William T. Holmes (1996, p. 2) elaborated on the intent and requirements of the California Hazards Reduction Act of 1986, which led to the drafting of Milestone 4 under Initiative 1.2.

The California Hazards Reduction Act of 1986 required the Seismic Safety Commission to develop a five-year program designed to significantly reduce statewide earthquake hazards by the end of the century. The Commission's document, *California at Risk . . . 1987 to 1992*, contained several initiatives, including one which addressed pre-Act hospital structures. Milestone 4 under this initiative recalled the Building Safety Board's 1983 recommendation for a program that would have all hospital buildings in compliance with the Act by the year 2020. This would require vacating, replacing or upgrading an existing facility (Holmes 1996).

3.1.8 Waypoint 8. In December 1990, OSHPD Responds to Milestone 4

In response to Milestone 4, in 1987, OSHPD contracted with the Applied Technology Council (ATC), a California-based not-for-profit research organization, to complete a statewide inventory of hospitals. The purpose of the inventory as presented in the report, ATC-23, was to provide OSHPD and other state agencies, including the Seismic Safety Commission, with an assessment of the survivability of the hospitals surveyed should earthquake-induced high intensity ground motions, geotechnical failures, or failure of utility services occur (Applied Technology Council 1990).

The survey was based on a cursory inspection of hospitals to determine the design date and primary type of structural system for each hospital building. It was completed with the voluntary cooperation of the acute care hospitals in the State. The inventory was completed in 1989 and published in 1990. Data from the survey were merged with the data from an earlier "Uplift Study" inventory (updated by ATC in 1989). The survey included all general acute care hospital buildings in California. The ATC found that more than half the acute care hospital buildings in use in 1990 were built before the 1973 legislation increased seismic design and construction standards. Of these, 413 were built in the 1950s, 626 in the 1960s, and 348 between 1970 and 1973.

ATC further concluded that normal replacement of the older buildings was occurring at a very slow pace. This is a key point in what eventually followed. What is perceived to be a particularly slow pace for those whose interest is enhanced seismic safety may not be perceived as a particularly slow pace for hospital owners and operators, especially when an individual hospital has served for so long and at least well enough given the hospital owner's financial situation and user needs.

The ATC report also concluded that many of the pre-1973 buildings were potentially hazardous to their occupants in a major earthquake. The survey provided extensive data on the seismic condition of nonstructural systems, as well as information about the likelihood that hospital buildings could be self-sustaining during the first days following a major earthquake.

Though the data base very likely represented a fairly accurate picture of the earthquake survivability of existing acute care hospitals, the information for specific hospital buildings was not based on in-depth engineering analysis and, consequently, was not intended as a basis for requiring specific corrective actions or setting priorities among actual buildings. The data were not identified with individual facilities or buildings since confidentiality had been promised in exchange for industry cooperation.

In December 1990, OSHPD issued its response to Milestone 4, *A Recommended Program to Seismically Strengthen Pre-Hospital Act Hospital Facilities.* It was sent to the Seismic Safety Commission near the end of 1990 (Holmes 1996). The report stated that upgrading pre-Hospital Act buildings (those built before 1973) could be accomplished by (1) emptying the buildings of all "essential" functions, (2) demolishing and/or replacing the buildings, or (3) seismically strengthening the buildings. The process would require cooperation, funding, and time to bring these pre-existing hospital buildings into compliance. The report went on to say that legislation would be necessary to put a plan into action and begin the orderly repair, reconstruction or replacement of hospital buildings not in conformance with the Hospital Facilities Seismic Safety Act of 1973. As described, OSHPD's program would emphasize the importance of hospitals remaining operational after an earthquake by establishing a deadline for all California hospitals to comply with the Hospital Facilities Seismic Safety Act. OSHPD's report outlined the provisions that would subsequently, and for the most part, be incorporated into SB 1953.

The recommended program consisted of an Evaluation and Planning Phase lasting 5 years, and an Implementation Phase lasting 30 years. During the Evaluation and Planning Phase, all buildings and all portions of hospital buildings constructed before March 7, 1973, would be examined by a licensed structural engineer to determine whether the building, including nonstructural elements, was capable of meeting the intent of Section 15000 of the Health and Safety Code. The evaluation would be based on a standardized procedure. Each hospital facility with pre-1973 buildings would be required to file a comprehensive plan for compliance. The compliance plan was to indicate the steps by which the hospital's owner intended to bring the facility into compliance and identify the phasing out or reconstruction of non-complying structures and utility systems, or outline steps for relocation of essential services to facilities that comply with current standards. The plan for compliance would have to be reviewed and approved by OSHPD.

The Implementation Phase would begin at the end of the 5-year Evaluation and Planning Phase. OSHPD would monitor implementation progress at each facility in accordance with the approved compliance plan. The report stated that the system for establishing compliance must be straightforward, applied consistently, and offer options for uses of buildings within the 30 year implementation period.

A numerical rating system was suggested for application to each building to determine its compliance deadline. Advocates of the numerical rating system wanted to incorporate some mechanism to avoid hard deadlines and to give hospital owners the freedom to reduce risk and thus extend deadlines for brick and mortar retrofit. It was suggested that the numerical rating system be based on site seismicity, estimated seismic performance characteristics of the structure, and the extent of hospital essential functions and/or hospital beds contained in the building. It was argued that the primary factor for determining compliance deadlines should be the structural evaluation, with the lowest rated buildings being assigned a deadline of about 10 years from the start of the program. It was suggested that the compliance deadline should be variable, determined at any time by the current values of the determinant factors. Thus, an owner could extend the compliance deadline of a building by removing essential functions or by improving projected seismic performance.

Finally, and very importantly, OSHPD recognized the importance of securing means for funding projects under the program. It suggested in the report that financial incentives and support would be necessary for some facilities if they were to realistically fulfill the steps outlined in their compliance plans. As we will see, the State Legislature did not include either financial incentives or financial support to healthcare organizations engaged in reconstruction or repair. The State was experiencing financial shortages and the legislature was apparently reluctant to underwrite the costs of implementing the program. This became a central factor in implementation problems that developed in the succeeding years. Hospital owners viewed the legislation as an unfunded mandate.

3.1.9 Waypoint 9. More Earthquakes

The Whittier Earthquake (1987) and Loma Prieta Earthquake (1989) each provided an opportunity to compare the seismic performance of hospital buildings built before and after the 1973 legislation. Very few hospitals were structurally damaged by the Loma Prieta Earthquake, perhaps because the location of the epicenter in the Santa Cruz Mountains did not "test" as many hospitals as an epicenter on the Hayward fault, which runs through heavily urbanized areas, might have. Nonstructural damage, however, was widespread. The Building Safety Board collected damage reports from hospital owners and design professionals and found that certain hospital components exhibited a high incidence of damage. These nonstructural components included emergency generators, elevators, communications systems, bulk oxygen tanks, and furniture, fixtures, supplies, and other building contents. The Building Safety Board developed a seismic checklist of nonstructural elements judged "exceptionally vulnerable" to seismic damage that OSHPD sent to all hospitals in the State.

The January 1994 Northridge Earthquake severely damaged several acute care hospital facilities. Eight of the 91 acute care hospitals in the Los Angeles region (9%) were evacuated. Six of the eight hospitals evacuated patients within 24 h. Five of these six hospitals cited nonstructural damage (e.g., loss of electrical power; water damage from burst pipes, fire sprinklers, and ruptured rooftop water tanks) as the main reason for evacuation; the sixth hospital cited both structural and nonstructural damage. The seventh hospital evacuated patients 3 days after the event, and the eighth hospital evacuated patients 2 weeks after the earthquake. These last two hospitals sustained nonstructural damage, but since it was not as extensive as that of the other six hospitals, they did not immediately evacuate patients. In the end, the decision to evacuate these two hospitals was based on delayed identification of structural damage, despite initial inspections by in-house personnel and local structural engineers who had found no damage. Nearly 1,100 patients were evacuated from the eight hospitals. Four of the eight hospitals that evacuated patients, including the two that did not evacuate immediately, were subsequently demolished (Schultz et al. 2003). More than $3 billion in hospital-related damages were attributed to the Northridge earthquake.

Shortly after the Northridge earthquake, OSHPD sent structural engineers, fire marshals, and construction advisors to assess the approximately 750 state-licensed facilities in the affected area. Within a week, approximately 400 facilities, including all significantly damaged sites, had been inspected. Nearly 95% of these were free of significant structural damage, although damage to nonstructural items such as storage shelving and equipment was widespread. There were no structural collapses. Structures, ranging in age from 24 to 68 years old (all built before 1973), were damaged most severely. In seven of the eight most damaged structures, failure occurred in nonductile concrete shear walls, characterized by severe diagonal cracking. In addition, there was significant damage to penthouse structures (walls and bracing) and roof-mounted equipment (Aurelius 1994).

3.2 Enacting SB 1953

It had become evident to seismic safety advocates that pre-1973 hospital buildings were not being withdrawn from use nearly quickly enough to meet their objectives. The effects of the Northridge Earthquake on hospitals provided all the additional incentive they needed to advance legislation addressing their concern about hospital buildings built before 1973. Within 2 weeks of the earthquake, California's State Assemblyman Margolin sent a memorandum to members of the legislature requesting co-authors of a bill he was authoring to require retrofit of existing hospitals, to toughen seismic safety standards, and to require the Department of Health Services to produce a report within 90 days on the causes of failure and the emergency preparedness of hospitals in the Los Angeles area.

On February 25, 1994, State Senator Alfred Alquist introduced a bill that had been drafted by the State Seismic Safety Commission staff and forwarded to him for his consideration and action. When enacted, the bill became known as SB 1953. SB 1953 was introduced into the California Senate only 5 weeks after the Northridge Earthquake. The early draft was amended half a dozen times through the spring and summer and passed the Assembly on August 29, 1994 and the Senate on August 30, 1994. The bill was signed into law in September by the governor as an amendment to the Hospital Facilities Seismic Safety Act of 1983.

Others, in addition to Assemblyman Margolin were anxious to spur action that would upgrade or replace pre-1973 hospitals. Senator Tom Hayden of Santa Monica introduced SB 878 on February 23, 1995, 13 months after the Northridge Earthquake and 6 months after Senator Alquist's bill had been signed into law. The legislation was introduced following the issuance of OSHPD's report on damages to pre-1973 hospitals, including two in Senator Hayden's district:

> . . The OSHPD report further finds that 23 pre-1973 health facilities were the most seriously damaged in the Northridge earthquake. Failure of pre-1973 buildings at St. John's Hospital and Health Center and other locations showed "... significant risk to the life safety of the occupants of older, unapproved hospital buildings" (California Senate Bill 878 1995, as introduced).

The legislation, if enacted, would have been much more draconian than Alquist's legislation. It called for completing retrofits or replacement of the pre-1973 hospitals within 3 years of the enactment of the legislation.

> All pre-1973 hospital buildings shall be upgraded or replaced to meet all applicable existing seismic safety building standards within three years of the effective date of the act that adds this article (California Senate Bill 878, 1995, as introduced).

The bill was voted down by a two-thirds vote in the Senate, but, with draft legislation such as this calling for the work to be completed within impossible deadlines, it is reasonable to conclude that the targeted agencies and the structural engineering, design, and construction industries were much more comfortable with the Alquist legislation and that the targeted hospital owners were of a similar mind.

3.3 Many Actors Were Involved in Shaping the Legislation

The preceding discussion may seem to imply a relatively rational, orderly, and sequential process for the development and enactment of SB 1953. That, however, is not exactly the case. The actual process that ultimately resulted in SB 1953 having been enacted was dynamic, iterative, and often characterized by conflict among various interests and perspectives. The process was similar to that of virtually all policymaking efforts that attempt to address a complex situation or set of issues that involves the differing interests and concerns of many actors. The many stakeholders lobbied for their interests while the bill was being drafted and considered, as well as after the law was enacted and the administrative regulations intended to implement SB 1953 were being developed.

Damaging earthquakes in California had led advocates of seismic safety to press for legislation to enhance safety and to create organizations in State government that would continue to focus on earthquake issues. SB 1953 was a result of efforts by the California Seismic Safety Commission, OSHPD, and the professional earthquake engineering community to require retrofit or replacement of pre-1973 hospital buildings. Proposals from seismic safety advocates were not considered, however, in a political vacuum. During the 8 month period between the introduction of the bill leading to SB 1953 and its enactment into law, healthcare organizations that would have to pay for the improvements were actively involved in trying to shape the legislation and later to shape the regulations that would be adopted to implement the policy. Some worked primarily through the California Healthcare Association (CHA), an association housed in Sacramento that represents the interests of healthcare organizations. In addition to the CHA efforts, Kaiser-Permanente, a large, vertically integrated HMO, was viewed by some as having significant influence on the outcome of SB 1953 because it was considered a model of how hospitals could be upgraded or replaced. Indeed, one element of a bill (SB 842) to provide relief to hospitals in compliance by 2008 while maintaining the spirit of SB 1953 was informally dubbed the "Kaiser plan". Kaiser is perhaps unique among West Coast healthcare organizations in that the millions of subscribers to its health insurance provide ongoing cash flow through payment of premiums, allowing for corporate strategic planning and an ability to invest in new or upgraded healthcare facilities. In another case, the Service Employees International Union (SEIU) supported SB 1953 as a workplace safety issue, pressing for an early timetable for reducing the likelihood of personal injury from structural and nonstructural failures in healthcare buildings.

All of the interested parties worked to affect the content of SB 1953, administrative regulations developed subsequently for implementing the legislation, and modifications to the regulations in the years following their adoption. Once the SB 1953 regulations were adopted, any changes would have to be made through processes established by the California Building Standards Law, which requires state agencies to submit any proposals for changing building standards to the State Building Standards Commission for adoption consideration during its annual code adoption cycle. Thus, amending the regulations to reflect the emerging retrofit design issues and problems is a time-consuming process, as the State Building Standards Commission can take as long as 24 months to approve any proposed changes.

SB 1953, its initial regulations, and subsequent legislation and regulatory changes were developed within a complex web of actors, institutions, and interests. The process would have been complex simply by virtue of the numerous interests involved. It was made more complex, however, because healthcare finances themselves were in turmoil during the process. Moreover, because California had adopted term limits for legislators, none of those who had created and debated the initial legislation was present later to help fix the problems that arose during implementation. Those who were in the legislature when adjustments were called for did not "own" the issue or the legislation and were understandably reluctant to tackle a complex issue fraught with conflict. After all, term limits meant that they had only a few years in office. They had their own agenda and they would not be around when compliance was scheduled to be completed. In short, the entire process was complex, took place in a dynamic environment, and was interlaced with conflict.

References

Applied Technology Center (ATC) (1990) ATC-23 General acute care hospital earthquake survivability inventory for California. Applied Technology Council, Redwood City

Aurelius E (ed) (1994) The January 17, 1994 Northridge, CA earthquake: summary report. EQE International, San Francisco

California Codes, Government Code (1974) Section (8870–8870.95) Seismic Safety Act Statutes

Castle RO, Alt J, Savage J, Balazs E (1974) Elevation changes preceding the San Fernando earthquake of February 9, 1971. Geology 2:61–66

Castle RO, Church JP, Elliott M (1976) A seismic up-lift in Southern California. Science 192:251–253

Geschwind C (2001) California earthquakes: science, risk and the politics of hazard mitigation. The John Hopkins University Press, Baltimore

Holmes WT (1996) The program for seismic rehabilitation of existing hospitals in California (Senate Bill 1953). In: CD RO: Proceedings of the Pan Pacific Hazards '96 Conference, Pan Pacific Hazards Conference, Vancouver

Lagorio HJ, Olson RA, Reitherman RB (1995) Charting the course for the future: the Alfred E. Alquist Hospital facilities Seismic Safety Act of 1983. Prepared for the Office of Statewide Health Planning and Development, Health and Welfare Agency, State of California by the Center for Environmental Design Research, University of California. University of California, Berkeley

Office of Statewide Health Planning and Development (2010) State of California. http://www.oshpd.ca.gov/FDD/About_Us/History/index.html

Poland CD (1994) Repair and retrofit of health care facilities. Earthq Spectra 10(1):113–123

Real CR, Bennett JH (1976) Palmdale bulge. Calif Geol 29:171–173

Schultz CH, Koenig KL, Lewis RJ (2003) Implications of hospital evacuation after the Northridge, California, earthquake. N Engl J Med 348:1349–1355

Seismic Safety Commission (1986) California at risk: reducing earthquake hazards 1987 to 1992. State of California, Sacramento

State of California, Hospital Safety Building Board (2003) Appeal procedures of the Hospital Building Safety Board. State of California, Sacramento. http://www.oshpd.cahwnet.gov/Boards/HBSB/board.pdf

State of California, California Statutes (1973) Hospital Facilities Seismic Safety Act of 1973 (Senate Bill 519). State of California, Sacaramento

State of California. Joint Commission on Seismic Safety (1974) SP 45: meeting the earthquake challenge. The final report to the legislature by the Joint Committee on Seismic Safety. State of California, Sacramento

State of California Senate (1969) Concurrent Resolution 128, California Statutes, 1969. Resolution Chap. 378, p 4080

Steinbrugge K, Schader E, Bigglestone H, Weers C (1971) San Fernando earthquake, February 9, 1971. Pacific Fire Rating Bureau, San Francisco, August 10

Chapter 4
SB 1953: The Law, the Program, and the Implementation Challenge

SB 1953 was introduced and enacted quickly following the Northridge Earthquake, but its basic elements had been developed over more than a decade before the earthquake. The legislature did not develop the law in haste in response to the Northridge Earthquake, nor was the law developed without substantial input from technical experts on building performance, State agencies, hospital owners, and others. SB 1953 is, essentially, a minor rewrite of OSHPD's response to the Milestone 4, Initiative 1.2 in the California Seismic Safety Commission's report entitled *A Recommended Program to Seismically Strengthen Pre-Hospital Act Hospital Facilities* (Seismic Safety Commission 1986). There is one noteworthy difference between what the Seismic Safety Commission and OSHPD proposed and what was finally enacted. Whereas both the Seismic Safety Commission and OSHPD indicated the need for some kind of financial assistance and flexible compliance methods for hospitals to meet the compliance deadlines, SB 1953 did not provide financial assistance, financial incentives, or compliance flexibility for hospitals to help them comply. It simply provided hard milestones for compliance without enabling funding or access to funding. This would prove to be a serious obstacle to implementation.

4.1 The Legislative Declaration

The legislative findings and declaration that introduce the legislation make clear the purposes for SB 1953. The legislative declaration reminds Californians of the vulnerability of hospitals in the Northridge Earthquake of January 17, 1994. Several hospitals built before the Alfred E. Alquist Hospital Facilities Seismic Safety Act of 1973 suffered major damage and had to be evacuated, but hospitals built to comply with the 1973 standards suffered very little structural damage, thus demonstrating the effectiveness of the Act. However, both pre and post-Act hospital facilities suffered nonstructural damage that "prevented hospitals from being operational, caused the loss of one life, triggered evacuations, unacceptable property losses, and added

D.J. Alesch et al., *Natural Hazard Mitigation Policy: Implementation, Organizational Choice, and Contextual Dynamics*, Environmental Hazards, DOI 10.1007/978-94-007-2235-4_4, © Springer Science+Business Media B.V. 2012

additional concerns on emergency medical response" (California State Senate SB 1953, 1994).

The legislative declaration cited the 1989 survey conducted by the Applied Technology Council (ATC) for OSHPD, saying that it indicated "over 83% of the state's hospital beds were in buildings that did not comply with the Alfred E. Alquist Hospital Facilities Seismic Safety Act because they were issued permits prior to the effective date of the Act. Furthermore, 26% of the beds are in buildings posing significant risks of loss of life and hospital functionality because they were built before modern earthquake codes." The statute, as enacted, states that "the older hospitals pose significant threats of collapse in major earthquakes and loss of functions in small or more distant earthquakes" (California State Senate SB 1953, 1994). The legislation quotes the ATC report as saying:

> . . . of the 490 hospitals surveyed, nine are in Alquist-Priolo Earthquake Fault Rupture Zones, 31 are in areas subject to soil liquefaction, 14 in areas with landslide potential, 33 in flood zones, and 29 have a possible loss or disruption of access (§15097.100).

4.2 The Substantive Content of SB 1953

SB 1953 states the means by which it intends that the situation be remedied with respect to hospitals built before the State imposed the 1973 standards and still tougher standards in 1983. It specified several critical dates. The first of these was June 30, 1996. By that time, OSHPD was to have developed definitions of earthquake performance categories for earthquake ground motions for both new and existing hospitals. The law indicates three levels of performance:

1. "Reasonably capable of providing services to the public after a disaster, designed and constructed to resist, insofar as practical, the forces generated by earthquakes . . ."
2. "In substantial compliance with the pre-1973 California Building Standards Codes, but not in substantial compliance with the regulations and standards developed by (OSHPD) pursuant to the Alfred E. Alquist Hospital Facilities Seismic Safety Act of 1983. These buildings may not be repairable or functional but will not significantly jeopardize life."
3. "Potentially at significant risk of collapse and that represent a danger to the public."

OSHPD was unable to comply with the date specified in the legislation for completing the program regulations. The agency was to have completed its program regulations by June 30, 1996. The regulations were not completed until March of 1998, probably because of the complexity of the problems and controversy about how to resolve the substantive issues involved in reviewing and commenting on the regulations.

The second critical date specified in the law was January 1, 2008. By that date, "any general acute care hospital building that is determined to be a potential risk of collapse or pose significant loss of life shall only be used for non-acute care hospital purposes." This implies that buildings judged to be within the most dangerous classification would have to be removed from acute care service, retrofitted, or replaced by that date. The law provided, however, that "a delay in this deadline may be granted by (OSHPD) upon a demonstration by the owner that compliance will result in a loss of health care capacity that may not be provided by other general acute care hospitals within a reasonable proximity" (§15097.127). The possibility of a delay in compliance was written into the regulations as a series of 1 year extensions up to 5 years.

The third critical date was January 1, 2030. By that date, all hospital buildings used for inpatient acute care would have to be brought into compliance with the Alfred E. Alquist Hospital Facilities Seismic Safety Act of 1983. SB 1953 gives hospital owners two fundamental options. "In accordance with the compliance schedule approved by (OSHPD), but in any case no later than January 1, 2030, owners of all acute care inpatient hospitals shall either:

- Demolish, replace, or change to non-acute care use all hospital buildings not in substantial compliance with the regulations and standards developed by (OSHPD) pursuant to the Alfred E. Alquist Hospital Facilities Seismic Safety Act and this act or
- Seismically retrofit all acute care inpatient hospital buildings so that they are in substantial compliance with the regulations and standards developed by (OSHPD) pursuant to the Alfred E. Alquist Hospital Facilities Seismic Safety Act and this act" (§15097.128).

Hospital owners who did not comply with the provisions of the Act were subject to severe penalties:

> Unless the hospital places its license in voluntary suspension, the state department (of Health) *shall* (emphasis added) suspend or refuse to renew the license of a hospital that has received a notice of violation from the office because of its failure to comply with either Section 15097.127 15097.128 (§15097.129).

Those hospitals with licenses that were suspended or not renewed could have that license reinstated or renewed by a written notice of compliance issues by OSHPD. SB 1953 also made noncompliance a criminal offense for hospital owners, consistent with the language included in all California bills involving local government (e.g., hospitals owned by county governments and special districts).

4.3 OSPHD'S SB 1953 Administrative Regulations

Enacting legislation is usually only the first step in developing regulatory policy. Administrative agencies are charged with developing the regulations that further define the policy and make it operational through one or more programs. The administrative rules usually have the force of law and, thus, are an integral part of the policy. Following enactment of SB 1953, OSHPD was required to devise program regulations, including defining and categorizing earthquake performance for the various types of structures, procedures for evaluating the likely structural and nonstructural seismic performance of individual facilities, and regulations for complying with the provisions of the law. OSHPD submitted its proposed regulations and procedures to the California Building Standards Commission and they were adopted on March 18, 1998. The task of developing the regulations and procedures involved a large number of organizations, each of which had a stake in the content of those rules. As one might expect, those stakeholders represented a wide array of values, goals, and priorities.

The Facilities Development Division (FDD) of OSHPD was and is the unit responsible for implementing the law. Its responsibilities included developing and implementing building regulations for all geotechnical, structural, mechanical, electrical, and fire-life safety matters. The FDD had a small staff and little time to develop the building design retrofit regulations within the approximately 2 years to meet the 1996 date for submitting its proposed code changes to the Building Standards Commission. Since the State Hospital Building Safety Board (HBSB) serves in an advisory capacity, the FDD looked to the HBSB for assistance. Representatives from the California Association of Hospitals and Health Systems (CAHHS) and the California Society for Hospital Engineering (CSHE) served as members of the HBSB. The CAHHS Health Facilities Task Force and the CSHE Codes Committee members served as a resource to the hospital representatives on the HBSB.

The HBSB appointed a Special Committee to work on the engineering aspects associated with retrofitting existing hospital structures and the requirements for the regulations necessary to implement the law. The Special Committee, on behalf of the HBSB, was to advise OSHPD on requirements for the regulations. In addition to OSHPD engineers, several prominent structural engineers and active members of the earthquake engineering community were named as committee members. The committee completed its work, but not without disagreement and discussion concerning alternative approaches. The report, FEMA 178, which was still in draft form at that time and on which much of the evaluative criteria for individual buildings was based, depended on engineering judgment concerning the seismic resistance of individual buildings. Anonymous participants in the committee deliberations said the OSHPD could not accept judgments as part of the pass-fail decision, even if the judgments were to be made by peer review panels. OSHPD called for standards consisting of documentable certainty not augmented by judgment to come up with pass-fail interpretations.

4.3.1 Concerns with Both Structural and Nonstructural Performance

It is important to understand that the SB 1953 program regulations addressed both 'structural' performance and 'nonstructural' performance. Acute care hospital buildings, if they were to remain functional following a significant earthquake, required that both structural and nonstructural building components remained operable.

Structural performance has to do with how the building itself responds to seismic forces. In simplified terms, seismic forces include shaking and ground movement. Most of us think of gravity as the primary force on buildings, but earthquakes generate horizontal ground motion typically represented as a percent of the force of gravity. In earthquake country, structural engineers have been active participants in creating building designs that are engineered to resist earthquake forces. A key role of structural engineers is to ensure that the building (or other structure) is designed to withstand various levels of earthquake forces. No building is earthquake proof, but buildings can be designed to withstand modest earthquakes with no resulting damage and moderate events with little or no damage. This, of course, is not the only reason for the participation of structural engineers in designing buildings. For many decades, structural engineers have been active participants in building design regardless of whether the buildings were expected to be subjected to earthquakes. Structural engineers design for natural forces including gravity and wind as well as earthquakes. Most hospital buildings in the California inventory had structural engineers involved in the design.

In general, the guidelines adopted for the SB 1953 program emerged from evaluations of various weaknesses in buildings based on their performance in past earthquakes. Based on the evaluation results, buildings were to be assigned a Seismic Performance Category (SPC) with SPC-1 rated buildings classified as posing the most significant risk of collapse and to life safety.

OSHPD required that, where possible, its SB 1953 regulations for structural performance would follow model codes and national standards. National guidelines were considered important because they were considered "consensus documents" developed by the professions. "Consensus documents" are those that have been subjected to extensive review by the earthquake engineering profession and for which a general agreement has been reached on the contents. Not surprisingly, members of the earthquake engineering profession actively supported using the national guidelines as the basis for the regulations. The Special Committee chose to utilize the Federal government's 1992 NEHRP (National Earthquake Hazard Reduction Program) guidelines for *The Seismic Evaluation of Existing Structures: FEMA 178* (Federal Emergency Management Agency 1992) as a basis for its criteria to rate hospital buildings.

Nonstructural features of a building include those things within and appurtenant to the building that make the building functional for the use intended, but that are not integral to the performance of the structure itself. Nonstructural features include suspended ceilings, pipes carrying gasses and water, electrical wiring and lighting, book cases and other kinds of equipment, and so forth. Damage to nonstructural elements can, of course, reduce significantly the capacity of a building to be used for its primary functions, such as healthcare. Falling equipment, failed exit signs, and ruptured pipes can also result in injuries or death. SB 1953 was intended to address both structural and nonstructural seismic concerns.

4.3.2 Regulations Developed in the Context of Some Ambiguity

Developing the set of regulations that would convert SB 1953 from a legislative policy into a program was anything but easy. One important area of discussion, if not conflict, was defining the basic criteria for what constituted an unsafe acute care hospital building. Life safety generally means that, during an earthquake, a structure should perform sufficiently well that those inside the building will not die as a consequence and that they should be able to exit the building safely. The general intent of those working on and reviewing the regulations was that an acute care hospital building should be safe to exit in the event of an earthquake and should not come down in the next good-sized aftershock. The difficulty came in attempting to specify exactly what that meant in objective, quantifiable terms.

The program regulations for the SB 1953 program relied heavily on FEMA 178, which concerned itself with life safety. The law, however, did not address life safety; it addressed "collapse." The standard of "collapse" is less stringent than the standards for "life safety" and, unfortunately, the structural engineering community had no evaluation method that addressed collapse until much later in the SB 1953 story. Participants in the process told us that some structural engineering practitioners suspected they would get into trouble with a "Life Safety" criterion because it brought into consideration every possibility of threats to life, no matter how remote or even whether the perceived deficiency had never caused injury in the past. Thus, the issue became how to address the dictate of the law (collapse) when the only available standard evaluation methods were for life safety. FEMA 273 would provide additional insights when completed in October 1997, but being only partially completed when the regulations were being developed, it was of limited use (Federal Emergency Management Agency 1997).

The NEHRP *Guidelines for Seismic Rehabilitation of Buildings* (FEMA Publication 273) was in draft stages at the time the regulations were being developed. Had it been completed, it would have provided an alternative means, but not the only means, for evaluating the seismic resistance of buildings. Thus, those who were writing the program requirements and those who were reviewing and commented on those regulations relied heavily on FEMA 178 (Federal Emergency Management Agency 1992) as the basic guideline for the SB 1953 regulations. In the absence of a completed, peer reviewed consensus document on which to rely (i.e., FEMA 273), there were no specific criteria or rules on how to determine a life safety standard. Nor were there easy ways to measure or identify a "margin against collapse" or of what would constitute a risk of life-threatening damage. As one might expect, issues arose about what constituted the appropriate standards for life safety.

While preventing collapse was a performance measure that could be assessed objectively using professional engineering knowledge; life safety was perceived by many as an ambiguous requirement. This led to a simplification of the regulations: an evaluation approach was selected that equated life safety with collapse prevention. There is no definition of life safety in Article 1 of Chap. 6 of the SB

1953 regulations. A partial reference to life safety occurs in the definition of SPC 2: "These buildings do not significantly jeopardize life…" It is possible that this definition caused confusion in the OSHPD's implementation of the law. It was not phrased in terms of a loss of significant numbers of lives such as would be expected in a collapse. It could be interpreted as a significant risk to a life, a much higher standard than prevention of collapse. This caused a lot of concern among engineering practitioners about falling hazards in buildings that could strike a person or two but would not necessarily kill many people. It is not necessary that the building be unusable after the earthquake for people to be killed in it. People can be killed within a building even if it does not collapse during the quake. Illustratively, if ceramic tiles are shaken loose and crash down in a stairwell, people are likely to be injured or killed. Exposure to electrical wiring or broken gas pipes can also kill people in a building that remains standing.

However, the difficulty of creating an operational definition or what constitutes life safety in the context of SPC 2 seems to have led rule makers to use structural collapse prevention as the surrogate for life safety. Importantly, this resulted in more restrictive regulations that became the primary basis for the structural performance categories used in the assessment of the pre-1973 hospital buildings, as well as the determination of what would be required to meet the requirements of SB 1953. The dilemma led OSHPD into a series of decisions about the NPC 2, SPC 1-2, NPC3 definitions that were all basically conservative and, in the minds of some practitioners we interviewed, excessive. The matter was not resolved until years later when a completely different approach to evaluation was adopted.

Based on our discussions with many of the individuals engaged in developing or reviewing and commenting on the regulations, we concluded that the major stakeholders involved in the development of the regulations did not fully anticipate the many issues that would arise during implementation. The specific performance period set forth in the law created a relatively small window for OSHPD to prepare the regulations, thereby limiting time to evaluate fully the impact of the proposed regulations and to gain the necessary consensus for retrofit guidelines for hospitals. Thus, the regulations can be seen as having been devised under the constraint of limited knowledge and experience in the retrofit of complex structures and systems, and under a significant degree of ambiguity due to the lack of a specific standard on life safety. Further, according to some stakeholders, it appeared that the process of developing the regulations was conditioned by attorneys from the regulatory agency (OSHPD), which eventually resulted in the regulations becoming very conservative.

Having drafted the regulations, one last step remained before OSHPD could begin implementing the program. In the State of California, it is the Building Standards Commission, governed by the Section 18930 of the Administrative Procedure Act of the State of California, that bears responsibility for adopting and publishing all State building regulations. The Commission includes 11 members, most of whom have technical backgrounds (e.g., architects, engineers, fire officials). The Commission has five committees, one of which handles the adoption of hospital building regulations. As a part of the adoption process, the Commission holds public hearings to review proposed new requirements and amendments to building regulations. While final regulations must be published within 180 days after adoption, there is a provision that emergency issues require publication within 30 days of filing.

Development of SB 1953-mandated building regulations had begun with identifying and selecting applicable model codes and national guidelines to be used as the principal source documents. The model codes and guidelines were applied as necessary to meet the legislative mandate. The regulations were developed in an open forum by OSHPD and were reviewed by the Hospital Building Safety Board acting as an outside advisory group. In the case of SB 1953, due to the complexity of the issues, OSHPD used the resources of a special committee appointed by the Hospital Building Safety Board to aid in developing the regulations. When completed, the regulations went through the California Building Standards Commission's adoption process, which included technical review and public comment. At the conclusion of this process, in 1998, the regulations were published as the official regulations interpreting the law and governing the program.

In retrospect, it seems that as the design community gained experience applying the regulations and became acquainted with the actual problems of seismic retrofitting acute care hospitals, that the regulations would benefit from amendments reflecting the knowledge gained. Still, when recommended modifications were submitted to the State's regulatory review and adoption, up to 2 years were required to make changes. This was viewed as unacceptable by the hospitals, given the stringent and short deadlines specified in SB 1953. An initiative by the California Hospital Association, supported by the Seismic Safety Commission and other stakeholders, resulted in a legislative change requiring that any amendments to the SB 1953 regulations submitted to the Building Standards Commission would be considered "emergency regulations" requiring action in only 6 months.

Even though the time between enactment of the law (January 1995) and the requirement of adoption of the regulations (March 1998) was considered by many to be a very short period for developing such a complex set of regulations and procedures, OSHPD staffers believed "a rational and realistic solution to the seismic mitigation problem for hospital buildings" including prioritizing mitigation and replacement could be accomplished (Tokas and Schaefer 1999, p. 4). According to Tokas and Schaefer, the principal steps required for each noncompliant hospital were:

- Determine the seismic deficiencies of each hospital building;
- Mitigate nonstructural items that are required for a safe and orderly evacuation of the building as well as those required for maintaining *critical* functions of the hospital for patient care;
- Determine a level of structural strengthening based on life safety concerns and the economic benefits, schedule the structural strengthening at a time that other collateral deficiencies can be corrected; and
- Correct the deficiencies in the architectural systems to be upgraded within the normal remodel process.

4.4 The Time Line

OSHPD's regulations established dates by which each acute care hospital building was to comply with standards. The intent was to deal with the most critical threats to life safety and continued operations first and, then, by 2030, to bring all hospital facilities up to contemporary standards.

- *January 1, 2001.* This was the first critical date in the implementation schedule. By then, hospital owners were to have completed and submitted a seismic assessment of each building in which acute inpatient care was provided on that date. If the buildings did not meet current standards (did not comply with the Hospital Facilities Seismic Safety Act of 1973, as amended), the owner was to prepare and submit a plan for achieving compliance. This could be accomplished by removing the building from acute care inpatient service, performing seismic retrofit, or demolishing and rebuilding the structure.
- *January 1, 2002.* All acute care inpatient hospitals were to have met minimum equipment anchorage standards for specified nonstructural systems, including, for safe and orderly evacuation, emergency lighting, emergency power and emergency communications.
- *January 1, 2008.* All acute inpatient hospital buildings still classified as SPC-1 were to be taken out of service as acute care facilities.
- *January 1, 2030.* All acute inpatient hospital buildings were to have met the standards of the Hospital Facilities Seismic Safety Act of 1973 as amended. Failure to do so could result in loss of license.

4.5 Structural Performance Categories

The published administrative regulations created two sets of seismic performance categories for acute care hospitals. One of the two was a set of Structural Performance Categories (SPCs). All hospital buildings in the State were to be classified into one of five SPC ratings. Six categories were ultimately defined, with the first (SPC-0) being a default category (not actually in the legislation, but created for administrative convenience) for buildings for which no evaluation was submitted. Hospital owners were required to obtain sufficient professional assistance (typically from a structural engineer) to classify their individual buildings and to report their evaluations to OSHPD by January 1, 2001. A description of each category follows, along with the number of hospitals fitting each category as of 2002 (see Fig. 4.1) (Schaefer 2004).

- **SPC-0.** The legislation has no provisions for categorizing hospital buildings for which no seismic evaluation was submitted. Buildings in this category were assumed to be self-declared as non-complying and, in OSHPD reports were grouped as SPC 0, presumably for the sake of convenience. Of the 2,709 buildings, 73 fell into this categorization.

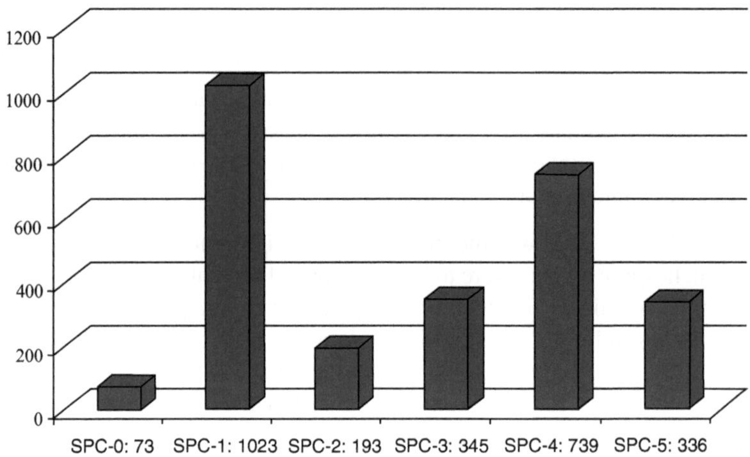

Fig. 4.1 Number of hospital buildings in each of five Structural Performance Categories (SPC) [2002] (Source: Facilities Development Division, California Office of Statewide Health Planning and Development. Presentation at MCEER Forum: Vision of Leaders (2004))

- **SPC-1.** These are buildings thought to pose a significant risk to the public. They were built before the 1973 standards were enacted. The newest of them was 25 years old when the regulations were completed. The regulations required that they be retrofitted, removed from acute care use, or replaced by January 2008. About 38% of all hospital buildings, or 1,023, were classified as SPC-1. Many of these were self-declared SPC-1, meaning that the designation was not determined by structural engineer's evaluation. Thus, it is difficult to say how many of these truly constituted hazards to life safety, although most probably did.
- **SPC-2.** These buildings were judged not to pose a significant risk of loss of life in the event of an earthquake, but they are potentially not repairable or functional after a major earthquake. They must be brought into compliance with the amended Alquist Act by January 1, 2030 or removed from acute care use. One hundred and ninety-three hospital buildings were declared SPC-2.
- **SPC-3.** These are hospital buildings in compliance with the Alquist Act. This category was intended to identify Steel Moment Resisting Frame buildings, designed and constructed in high seismic intensity areas prior to 1995. It was not intended to suggest that these buildings were better or worse than buildings classified as SPC 4; i.e., other hospital buildings constructed after 1973 but before 1989. This may have caused confusion among owners because many inferred that a building classified as SPC 3 was worse than a building classified as SPC 4 and that both were inferior to a building classified as SPC 5. Buildings classified as SPC 3 may be damaged in a major earthquake, but can be used beyond 2030, provided any damage is repaired to standards. Three hundred and forty-five buildings were classified as SPC-3.
- **SPC-4.** These are buildings in compliance with the Alquist Act. They may be damaged in a major earthquake and become temporarily unavailable, but they

can be used beyond 2030. Of California's 2,709 hospital buildings, 739 were classified SPC-4.

- **SPC-5.** These are buildings in compliance with the Alquist Act. They should be capable of providing service to the public after a major earthquake and can be used beyond 2030. Of California's 2,709 hospital buildings, 336 were classified SPC-5.

Using the definitions adopted for use in SB 1953, more than 40% of the acute care hospital buildings in California were deemed to pose a significant risk of collapse and public danger. Only about 12% were classified as being capable of providing service to the public after a major earthquake (SPC-5) and available for use beyond 2030. Many hospital buildings classified as SPC-3 and SPC-4 continued to provide services after the Northridge Earthquake in spite of the damage they incurred. Northridge Medical Center is one example of a hospital near the epicenter of that earthquake that was damaged but remained functional after the event.

4.6 Nonstructural Performance Categories

The second set of standards developed by OSHPD had to do with the performance of nonstructural elements of hospital buildings. Failure of nonstructural elements of hospital buildings during earthquakes was far more widespread than structural failure, and it created significant problems for providing continuing service immediately following an event. Five Nonstructural Performance Categories (NPC), were defined in addition to the default category of SPC-0. A description of each category follows. The number of hospitals fitting each category as of 2002 (Schaefer 2004) is shown in Fig. 4.2.

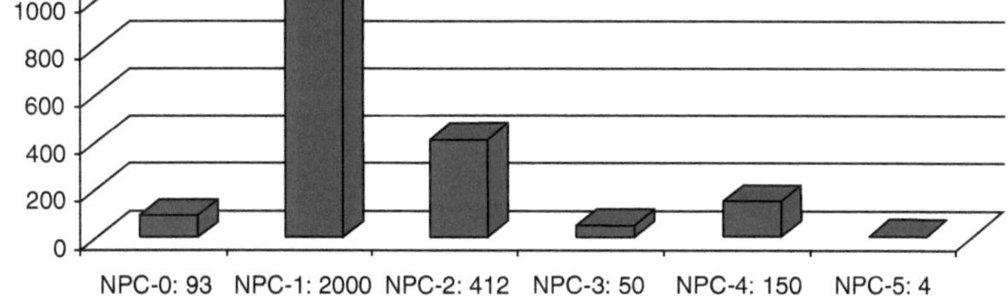

Fig. 4.2 Number of Acute Care Hospital buildings in each of five Nonstructural Performance Categories (NPC) [2002] (Source: Facilities Development Division, California Office of Statewide Health Planning and Development. Presentation at MCEER Forum: Vision of Leaders (2004))

- NPC-0. Buildings for which evaluations were not received and that are presumed to fall into the NPC-1 category. Ninety-three buildings of a possible 2,709 fit into this category. There is no formal classification of NPC-0; it is a convenient way used by OSHPD to categorize buildings for which no response was received.
- NPC-1. Buildings with systems not adequately anchored and braced. About 74% of all hospital buildings, or 2,000, were classified as NPC-1.
- NPC-2. Buildings with systems adequately anchored and braced for the safe evacuation of occupants, but not for continuous operation or even for speedy recovery. Four hundred and twelve hospital buildings were declared NPC-2.
- NPC-3. Buildings that meet NPC-2 requirements, but that also have selected systems that are adequately anchored and braced. All acute care hospitals are to meet this standard by 2008. Fifty hospital buildings were declared NPC-3.
- NPC-4. Buildings that meet NPC-3 requirements, and, in addition, all systems and areas are adequately anchored and braced. All acute care hospitals are to meet this standard by 2030. In 2001, fewer than 6% (150) of California hospitals met the standard.
- NPC-5. Buildings that meet NPC-4 requirements and on-site requirements for 72-h operation after a major earthquake. All hospital campuses are to meet these requirements by 2030, but as of the 2001 evaluation, only about 0.1% (4) of the buildings met them.

4.7 A Massive Job and a Tight Timetable

The implementation timetable for SB 1953 at the time thc program regulations were adopted by the California Building Standards Commission in 1998 was straightforward. First, hospital owners were to evaluate and report to the Office of Statewide Healthcare Planning and Development (OSHPD) the status of their facilities' structural and non-structural seismic resistance by January 2001. Second, the Act required that all acute care hospital facilities not in compliance with critical non-structural seismic safety standards bring communication, emergency systems, fire alarms, and emergency lighting in exit corridors up to contemporary standards by January 1, 2002. Third, acute care hospital facilities classified as SPC-1 were to be retrofitted or taken of service as acute care facilities by 2008 and replaced by 2030. All nonstructural systems not meeting state standards must be brought up to date by 2030 as well. Frequently, however, regulatory mandates are challenged and often modified in the context of factors and forces that become apparent during implementation. SB 1953 was no different.

The consequences of not complying with the SB1953 program could be severe. Owners of acute care, inpatient hospital facilities would have to comply with the terms of the act or possibly lose their hospital license. It was clearly stated in the legislation that the State shall suspend or revoke the hospital's license if it did not comply, but it was not clear to some of those who read the law that this was mandated. Some hospital owners and operators questioned whether the State would truly take away their license. Fewer than 100 owners of acute care inpatient hospitals failed to comply with the first SB 1953 deadline, January 1, 2001, by either self-declaring noncompliance of their facilities or having been determined to be non-compliant following an evaluation by a structural engineer. However, responses to subsequent deadlines by individual hospitals ranged from total compliance to virtually no compliance.

SB 1953 was enacted on the basis of assumptions and premises developed over a number of years. The statewide inventory of hospitals, conducted by the Applied Technology Council (ATC) at the behest of the California Seismic Safety Commission and published in 1990, was an approximation of the survivability of the hospitals surveyed should earthquake-induced high intensity ground motion, geotechnical failures, or failure of utility services occur (ATC 1990). The ATC survey provided extensive data on the seismic condition of nonstructural systems and information about the likelihood that hospital buildings could be self-sustaining during the first days following a major earthquake. The information for specific hospital buildings was not based on in-depth engineering analysis and was not intended as a basis for requiring specific corrective actions or setting priorities among actual buildings. The Commission had concluded from the ATC data that about 10% of the State's hospitals posed an imminent threat from a moderate earthquake (Tobin 2004).

However, the SB 1953 regulations were subsequently written in such a way that almost four times as many acute care hospital facilities were classified as at risk of imminent collapse from an earthquake. Indeed, the 2001 assessment of acute care hospital facilities required by OSHPD as the first step in implementing SB 1953 resulted in 38% (1027) of the facilities classified as SPC-1, posing serious threats to life. These buildings were to be repaired, replaced, or abandoned as acute care facilities by 2008. Another 78 buildings were not reported and were assumed to be SPC-1 buildings not in compliance with contemporary standards.

Three-fourths of the acute care hospital buildings, according to the 2001 assessment, had inadequate *nonstructural* elements. Some claimed that the number was so high because OSHPD employed "overly zealous interpretations of what met standards," but that, of course, was a matter of judgment. The hospitals that failed the nonstructural evaluation were to be brought into initial compliance of the most critical systems by January 2002, only a year after having been so classified. Only four acute care hospitals in the State were judged to be capable of providing all nonstructural services following a major earthquake. OSHPD reported that 608 of the facilities classified as SPC-1 were in the areas of California with the highest projected Peak Ground Acceleration (PGA) from earthquakes. These areas include the most heavily populated areas of the state, including the San Francisco Bay and greater Los Angeles metropolitan areas.

It became immediately obvious to those involved with the hospital industry and with hospital regulation that the job ahead was enormous. If the program were implemented on schedule, the number of hospitals that would have to be repaired or replaced in the 7 years from 2001 to 2008 was staggering: 1,100 hospital facilities would have to be retrofitted, taken out of service, or replaced and about 96% of the acute care inpatient hospital facilities in the State would have to be modified to meet nonstructural standards. For hospital owners whose buildings were classified as SPC-1, work on retrofit or replacement would have to begin essentially immediately.

If all that were necessary was to build anew or repair existing structures, the job would be almost impossible Plans would have to be formulated for the structure or structures, funding would have to be arranged, space for the facilities would have to be found or acquired in the case of rebuilding, plans would have to be submitted to OSHPD for review and approval before bids were let, contracts had to be awarded, and the facility built and prepared for occupancy within 7 years. Anyone who has experience with designing and building large, complex facilities requiring review and approval by a state agency knows that a 7 year timeframe is often minimal and quickly becomes inadequate in the event of contingent events. Going through this with more than 1,000 hospital buildings would, presumably, strain even California's inventory of structural engineers and construction firms. The challenge was daunting from the start.

No clear line distinguishes buildings that are likely to fail from those that are likely to survive earthquake forces. A great deal depends, of course, on the definition of the level of earthquake forces against which the facility must be resistant. There are uncertainties as to the resistance of individual existing facilities against earthquake forces. Until the Northridge Earthquake in 1994, for example, welded steel buildings were considered to be secure against all but the strongest earthquakes. However, following that earthquake, it was learned that steel welds failed in a significant number of buildings and, while none of those buildings collapsed, many were in need of expensive repairs. The uncertainties associated with seismic resistance creates a large gray area within which even very good structural engineers might disagree among themselves as to whether a specific structure may survive a particular event.

Some buildings, however, are not in the gray range and an assemblage of structural engineers would generally concur that the building would fail to survive specified forces. In a presentation on performance based engineering at the 2004 National Earthquake Conference, Chris Poland, a distinguished California structural engineer and past member of the Hospital Building Safety Board, stressed that regulatory bodies could achieve quick gains in the reduction of the risk from earthquakes by first classifying the buildings to be retrofitted in terms of those most likely to experience a catastrophic failure in the event of an earthquake and then focusing on fixing those problems first. That is, relevant parties could prioritize the buildings needing retrofit based on risk, correct the most serious problems immediately, and not get bogged down trying to do all buildings at once on a very tight deadline. By all accounts, this was the approach desired by those who drafted and supported SB 1953 (Tobin 2004). Proponents understood that trying to tackle all of the buildings at once would likely lead to a form of gridlock where little would be done. Importantly, and as stated previously, it appears that proponents were expecting that only about 10% of the State's hospitals would fit into the "most at risk" category. In retrospect proponents underestimated the amount of work that would need to be done, at least given the metrics that were eventually applied.

As always, the technical challenge was where to draw the line. In the case of SB 1953 regulations, some healthcare organizations and structural engineers argue that the SPC-1 threshold was set too high; that too many buildings were included in the imminent threat category. They argue that there should have been a clearer set of priorities so that the most dangerous buildings would have the most urgent timetable for addressing the problem. Supporters of the regulations argue that the line had to be drawn somewhere and that it was drawn appropriately in this case. In any event, the result of initial structural certification was that almost 40% of California's acute care hospitals were classified as being imminent threats to life safety in an earthquake and to continued functionality after the event. The Seismic Safety Commission recognized the need for clarification in this area when in its 2001 document, *Hospital Seismic Safety Findings and Recommendations*. It stated that the SPC-1 category should be refined to be consistent with risk levels, especially when extensions of time for compliance are requested (California Seismic Safety Commission 2001).

OSHPD's regulations required a site specific earthquake hazard assessment (Article 2.1.1) and specific building vulnerability analysis (Articles 2.4.3 and Articles 3, 4, and 5). Unfortunately, the contents of that analysis were based on FEMA 178 and, in this process, a large number of questions had to be answered and justified by analysis. Each question had equal importance in this evaluation. Failing one question automatically failed the building, whether that question truly represented a life-safety concern or not. The recommendations in Milestone 4 (see Chap. 3) were closer to a risk assessment than to a pass/fail regulation, but that recommendation was not integrated into the final regulations. Structural engineers had the option in the SB 1953 regulations (Article 2.7 Alternative Analysis) to employ advanced analysis on individual buildings. However, according to a knowledgeable practicing engineer, this required getting approval by OSHPD of the proposed methodology, which was a very time consuming and uncertain path to take. In general, hospital owners chose not to spend scarce resources to do this analysis, perhaps because they believed it would not be likely make any difference in the outcome: i.e., their facility would still be classified as SPC 1. In retrospect, the large number of hospitals requiring retrofit or replacement by 2008 ultimately became a significant administrative and political problem.

References

California Seismic Safety Commission (2001) Findings and recommendations on hospital seismic safety. State of California, Sacramento, November 2001

California State Senate SB 1953 (1994) Chaptered, 9 Sept 1994

Federal Emergency Management Agency (1992) NEHRP handbook for seismic evaluation of existing buildings: FEMA 178. FEMA, Washington, DC

Federal Emergency Management Agency (1997) NEHRP guidelines for the seismic rehabilitation of buildings: FEMA 273. FEMA, Washington, DC

Schaefer KA (2004) Earthquake resistant and resilient hospitals. Presented at visions of leaders: structural and geotechnical earthquake engineering research needs for the mitigation of earthquake risks for the next decade, MCEER Forum, September. http://mceer.buffalo.edu/research/nees/grandopen/Forum/schaefer.pdf.

Seismic Safety Commission (1986) California at risk: reducing earthquake hazards 1987 to 1992. State of California, Sacramento

Tobin T (2004) Personal communication

Tokas CV, Schaefer K (1999) The seismic safety program for hospital buildings in California, Part 2: the seismic retrofit program for existing California hospitals. In: Proceedings of the workshop design and retrofitting of hospitals, Palazzo Panchiatichi, Florence, Italy, 21–22 Oct 1999

Chapter 5
Implementing SB 1953: 1998 into 2005

California's hospitals are incredibly diverse. The list of owners includes not-for-profit organizations, investor-owned companies, general purpose local governments, special hospital districts, and agencies of the State, including universities. Some have a single, free-standing facility, but many consist of one or more campuses, each with multiple buildings. Some hospital owners own many facilities in different locations. Some have single buildings to which additions have been made over decades. Others consist of a single building without major renovations or additions.

Given the diversity of hospitals and their owners, the great variations in their financial circumstances, and the high costs of complying with SB 1953, one could hardly expect a uniform response by hospital owners whose facilities were classified as SPC-1. Indeed, the hospital owners' responses were many and varied, depending on the circumstances within which each of them found themselves when the SB 1953 regulations were promulgated and during the early years of program implementation.[1]

5.1 Continually Escalating Costs of Compliance

The estimates of how much it will cost hospital owners to comply with all the provisions of SB 1953 have grown almost astronomically since the program was enacted. "Initially, the cost of complying with SB 1953 was estimated at $14 billion statewide by 2030. However, the specific regulations of the law were not finalized

[1]The financial condition of hospitals and the major upheaval in healthcare economics is discussed in depth in Part III where we consider how owners and administrators made choices about whether or how to comply with SB 1953. It is impossible, however, to discuss the early years of implementation without some references to the severe financial problems of hospitals at the time the law was enacted, but we have tried to minimize the redundancy.

D.J. Alesch et al., *Natural Hazard Mitigation Policy: Implementation, Organizational Choice, and Contextual Dynamics*, Environmental Hazards,
DOI 10.1007/978-94-007-2235-4_5, © Springer Science+Business Media B.V. 2012

until a few years after the law's passage, and the estimate of compliance costs has grown to $24 billion – a sum equivalent to the total combined, undepreciated assets of all California hospitals" (University of California-Davis 2010). The total cost of complying with the structural and nonstructural requirements of SB 1953 will vary, of course, depending on how each healthcare organization responds.

In 2002, RAND, the non-profit, nonpartisan think tank headquartered in Santa Monica, California, produced a set of cost estimates for compliance that was commissioned by the California Healthcare Foundation. The RAND analysts concluded that meeting the initial requirements would cost about $42 billion. Meeting the nonstructural upgrade requirements for 2008 and 2030 would cost an additional $646 million (Meade et al. 2002). Since RAND's analysts were provided a reasonably reliable estimate of the number of square feet to be upgraded, the total cost varies up or down depending on the cost of structural and nonstructural retrofitting.

To estimate the cost of meeting SB 1953s structural requirements, RAND analysts created four basic scenarios. For the first of the four scenarios, the analysts used a nominal replacement cost of $1 million per bed, or about $666 per square foot. These replacement costs – representing the total out-of-pocket expenditures incurred in the process of complying with SB 1953 – were calculated using the actual costs associated with building and equipping several recently completed hospital projects (e.g., UCLA Westwood, UCLA Santa Monica, Sutter Roseville). Each scenario had a variant, "b", in which only 70% of the hospital beds were replaced. The 70% scenarios were predicated on a relatively low occupancy rate at the time of the analysis and population growth projections.

Scenario 1a assumed that all 41,100 beds in OSHPD's SPC-1 category would be replaced, for a total cost of about $41 billion. Scenario 1b, in which only 70% of the beds would be replaced, would cost about $28.8 billion. Scenario 2 subtracted the costs of medical furnishings and equipment from the total replacement cost to more closely approximate construction costs alone, yielding an assumed construction cost of $220 per square foot. Scenario 2 cost estimates were $8.8 billion for construction costs alone (Scenario 2a) and $6.2 billion for 70% replacement (Scenario 2b).

In Scenario 3, the analysts removed construction costs associated with parking structures (never part of SB 1953) and heating, ventilating, and air conditioning (HVAC). The rationale for these deletions was that parking structures contribute minimally to keeping a hospital operational after an earthquake, and that advanced HVAC systems could be viewed as medical equipment. Based on an assumed construction cost of $128 per square foot, Scenario 3 cost estimates were $5.1 billion (Scenario 3a) and $3.6 billion (Scenario 3b).

Finally, Scenario 4 was an attempt to isolate only those costs for facility replacement applied to seismic strengthening. In this way, the analysts were able to calculate what some might consider the "true" or "pure" costs of compliance with SB 1953. The RAND analysts used an estimate that seismic design elements add about 10–20% to the cost of a building's structural frame. Thus, the assumed construction costs were increased by about $3 per square foot. In that case, Scenario 4 projected costs in the area of $120 million for complete bed replacement (Scenario 4a) and $80 million to replace 70% of the beds (Scenario 4b).

No matter how one might pare away or reallocate the costs of replacing the healthcare facilities among various purposes, it seemed pretty straightforward that, as of 2002, healthcare owners would have to find and spend on the order of $40 billion to meet the requirements of SB 1953 as devised and interpreted by OSHPD. It really does not matter whether some of the costs consisted of medical equipment. Nor does it matter that some of the costs will pay for nonstructural equipment; one cannot simply pick up an HVAC system and move it from an existing facility about to be demolished into a new one being built. For practical purposes, then, all related costs including soft costs (the owners' costs to hire a design team, pay fees, manage the process, and most importantly, the operational costs of relocation or disruption to services) must be included in any reasonable and meaningful total cost estimate.

5.2 A Broad Array of Responses, Depending on Circumstance

SB 1953 was signed into law September 21, 1994. The policy's administrative regulations were adopted a little more than 3 years later in March, 1998 by the California Building Standards Commission and, thus, became administrative law. In a little less than 3 years, by January 1, 2001, each hospital was to have completed and submitted a seismic assessment of each building it owned or operated in which acute inpatient care was provided. If the buildings did not comply with the Hospital Facilities Seismic Safety Act of 1973 as amended, the owner was to prepare and submit a plan for achieving compliance.

The first requirement of the law, reporting conditions of pre-1973 facilities, was due January 1, 2001. As healthcare organizations hired structural engineers to assess what it would take to comply with SB 1953, many owners and administrators were stunned to learn how much it would cost and the extent of the logistic complications associated with structural retrofitting and nonstructural changes.

To say that healthcare organizations' responses to SB 1953 varied across organizations and through time would be an understatement. Based on our discussions with more than a 100 hospital owners and operators, there existed an underlying sense among most hospital owners and administrators that they would try to comply, even though some hospitals were opposed to the legislation or to the timetable for compliance for a variety of reasons: "It's an unfunded mandate," "It's a full employment act for structural engineers," "We're not likely to see an earthquake of any meaningful size here in my lifetime," "Our buildings are not as susceptible to damage as suggested by SB 1953," and so on. No matter their objection, almost all agreed that they would seek to comply with SB 1953, because law-abiding behavior was part of their corporate mission and because they understood the need to address concerns about facility safety. Still, the initial responses to the SB 1953 mandates came down to the circumstances in which individual owners and operators found themselves when the rules came into effect. Those relatively few healthcare organizations with sufficient resources to comply sought to comply. Those in dire financial circumstances sometimes saw no hope of complying with the law. Likewise, those who saw no way to stay open while remodeling or rebuilding saw no hope of complying with the law. Those healthcare organizations that saw themselves as having long term viability and short term financial problems typically began developing strategies they hoped would enable them to ultimately cope with the financial upheaval and the legislative mandates.

Readers might expect that a healthcare organization's responses to the challenges imposed by the Act might differ depending on whether the organization is a government, a not-for-profit organization, or an investor-owned business. We did not undertake a systematic study to distinguish the nature of responses by kind of owner, but we did interview owners and managers of hospitals owned by governments, not-for-profit organizations, and private investors. On the basis of those discussions, we concluded that there were several ways one could array the organizational responses, but none was compelling or more powerful in helping us understand the responses more than the respective missions and the financial circumstances of the individual organization. In other words, the degree of compliance was not clearly correlated with the type of hospital. Non-profits and investor-owned hospitals, for example, were equally as likely to be planning compliance.

Having said that, it is nonetheless important to note that different kinds of owners had different options available to them when attempting to bring their facilities into compliance. Investor-owned hospitals cannot attempt to float a bond issue through a public referendum. By the same token, one should not expect a county or a special hospital district to sell or close their medical facilities and move to another community that might afford better business opportunities. Clearly, then, some differences in behavior can be attributed to who owns the facility.

A few hospital owners and administrators we interviewed simply chose to ignore the pending 2008 deadline. These were managers of not-for-profit community and investor-owned hospitals, typically small hospitals with only one or two facilities, who believed they had little or no hope of generating the kind of money required to either retrofit or replace their facilities. They chose to substitute hope for action, hoping that the state would be politically unable to withdraw their hospital's license for failing to comply with structural and nonstructural requirements or that something else would happen to keep them from having to comply or that would enable them to pay for the changes. In a few cases, the mood was one of outright defiance: "Just let them try to take away our license!"

5.2.1 Responding to the Challenge

At the same time SB 1953 and other forces (e.g., increasing population and changing technologies and medical practice) were pushing for a building boom, most hospitals found themselves unable to pay for such a boom (Catholic Health World 2003). Privately owned hospitals, whether investor-owned or not-for-profit, faced significant financial obstacles to complying with SB 1953. At the facility level, many were faced with operating losses and reserves that were wholly inadequate to cover the costs of retrofit. One hospital manager told us that the estimate for completing initial renovations and related construction on the many buildings comprising its facility was about $1.38 billion. Moreover, some concluded that it would be more efficient in many cases to build new, rather than retrofit and then build new for 2030. In addition, some faced what they saw as almost intractable logistical problems at specific locations whether building a new facility or retrofitting the old one. In any event, changes in medical practice, third party financial coverage, and the need for greater operating efficiency called for new hospital designs.

As one might expect, managers of investor-owned hospital organizations made decisions about whether and how to comply with SB 1953 largely in terms of their objective to providing a positive return to their investors by providing healthcare services. Individual facilities were evaluated in terms of the extent to which they met the criterion. Tenet Healthcare Corporation, for example, announced early in 2004 that it planned to sell nearly one-third of its hospitals, 19 of them in California. Tenet's Chief Executive Officer said that the restructuring would create a company with the potential for stronger performance over the long term (Vogt 2004). Both investor-owned and larger not-for-profit organizations sold some facilities, closed some facilities, and built some new ones in areas where they could reasonably expect to generate a profit or, in the case of the not-for-profits, a surplus.

It made sense for larger healthcare organizations to evaluate their various facilities and to decide where it made sense to make additional investments and where it did not. If a facility with few prospects for profitability could be sold to someone else, that would provide cash for making improvements in other facilities. If the noncomplying facilities could not be sold, those facilities would most likely be closed: logic suggests that sunk costs are no reason to hold on to an asset with no prospect of generating a profit. Investor-owned healthcare organizations could shed themselves of facilities that were not generating sufficient return and replace them with facilities located in high-end markets where they could provide services with acceptable financial margins. They might be able to "cherry pick" markets by acquiring facilities owned by organizations that were unable to finance the required improvements and were ready to sell.

Some healthcare organizations had sufficient resources to initiate efforts to comply with SB 1953. Most notable among these is Kaiser Permanente. The organization had humble beginnings during the Great Depression, grew during World War II, and, following the War, became a pioneer in developing pre-paid healthcare programs. In 2010, Kaiser Permanente had 8,570,000 health plan members in nine states and the District of Columbia (Kaiser 2010). It is vertically integrated, comprising the not-for-profit Kaiser Foundation Health Plan and Hospitals and the Permanente Medical Groups. Unlike traditional healthcare organizations, Kaiser Permanente's vertical integration provides a continuing cash flow, potentially enabling the organization to comply with SB 1953 more readily than most other not-for-profit hospital organizations. Premiums from health plan subscribers support the hospitals and medical groups and provide a strong financial base for this organization to work toward SB 1953 compliance. Kaiser's response was to build new hospitals rather than retrofit old ones.

5.2.2 Hospital Closures Attributed, at Least in Part, to SB 1953 Costs

In more than one conversation with hospital executives, we were reminded that the ultimate consequences associated with policies made for complex situations are sometimes contrary to the originators' intended purposes. This is generally known among analysts as "the law of unintended consequences." There are always unintended consequences of action taken. In the case of SB 1953, for example, we were confronted with a paradox: a law intended to ensure adequate medical care *after* an earthquake appears to have actually reduced the availability of hospital care both *before and after* an earthquake, at least for those individuals living in low income areas and having the least ability to afford adequate and routine medical care. In the case of hospital closures that might be attributed at least in part to SB 1953 because of inadequate financial resources to retrofit and/or rebuild the facilities, healthcare access in some communities was reduced. Importantly, since the hospital organizations most likely to have the least in terms of financial resources tend also to care for society's least financially able, hospital closures tend to disproportionately affect society's poor. In the end, the quest to ensure adequate access to healthcare after an earthquake appears to have yielded reduced access both before and after said earthquake.

In saying this, our intent is not to argue that hospitals should not be seismically sound. Rather, our intent is to identify and describe what we think is a very real and wholly unintended consequence of injecting the SB 1953 policy into a complex environment.

Twenty-three general acute care hospitals in California closed between 1995 and 2000, with most of them closing in 1998, the same year the SB 1953 regulations were adopted. In *California's Closed Hospitals, 1995–2000*, analysts attempted to assess the reasons for those closures (Nicholas C. Petris Center 2001). Financial factors dominated. Most hospitals in California were financially stressed during the period, but "As a group, the closed hospitals reported some of the worst financial indicators." The report notes, "While the state's hospitals have amassed debt" at nearly twice the national average and maintain thin operating margins, the closed hospitals show even lower margins and greater accumulation of debt. Further, each closed hospital "performed poorly in the 3 years prior to closure, with a dramatic decline in the last year before closing" (Nicholas C. Petris Center 2001, pp. 11–12). The report concludes that "retrofit requirements are likely to lead to additional closures in areas where the market is over saturated and margins and bed use are low" (Nicholas C. Petris Center 2001, pp. 11–12). In 2000, the president of the California Healthcare Association predicted that closures related to seismic retrofit requirements would range from 50 to 150 (cited in Nicholas C. Petris Center 2001, p. 14). For hospitals in difficult financial circumstances, SB 1953 might have been the straw that broke the camel's back.

Almost all the hospitals that closed were in urban areas. The Los Angeles area experienced the most closures. Together, the closed hospitals accounted for only about 3.6% of available hospital beds in the State. That is a small percentage statewide, but the closed hospitals tended to be concentrated in lower income urban areas. Two closures removed all hospital care within a 15 mile radius and, in two other cases, the radius without service was nearly 15 miles. Almost half the closed hospitals were investor-owned, although investor-owned hospitals made up about only one-third of hospitals during that period. For example, Tenet Healthcare Corporation closed five investor-owned facilities.

The sale of 19 California hospitals announced by Tenet Healthcare prompted Marcy Zwelling-Aamot, MD, Los Angeles County Medical Association president, to say she was concerned that Tenet would be unable to find buyers for all of the hospitals, leading some of them to close and contributing to what she describes as a crisis in health care in Los Angeles. "You can't mistake the idea that these hospitals might close," said Dr. Zwelling-Aamot, a specialist in internal medicine and critical care. "Tenet is a well-versed, well-greased Fortune 500 company. If they cannot make money in the health care marketplace, who is going to buy the hospital?" (Vogt 2004).

Tenet stated that one reason it sold California facilities was SB 1953. The organization's Chief Executive Officer said the 19 hospitals for sale in California would have required a $1.6 billion investment to meet SB 1953 provisions. The 17 California hospitals that Tenet planned to continue operating in California were estimated to cost less than $300 million to bring up to standards. A Tenet spokesman "scoffed at the suggestion that the company was selling the hospitals as a means of generating cash to offset legal costs or to pay for a settlement in one of its legal battles. He said the divestiture of all 27 hospitals is expected to generate total net proceeds of about $600 million, much of which will be in the form of tax benefits" (Vogt 2004).

In August 2004, Northridge Hospital Medical Center announced it would close its Sherman Way campus in the Van Nuys area of the San Fernando Valley (Los Angeles). This facility, owned by Catholic Healthcare Services West (CHW) housed the sixth and largest emergency room scheduled to close in Los Angeles County in a 14 month period. CHW owned another hospital in the Northridge area and, perhaps in a move to increase efficiency, decided to close one of them. *The New York Times* reported that the announcement followed "by a week the closing of the emergency room at Elastar Community Hospital in the East Los Angeles neighborhood. In the last 2 years, four other emergency rooms, mostly in low-income areas, have closed in the county, primarily because of the high cost of treating thousands of uninsured people" (Madigan 2004).

The *Times* reported that a hospital spokesperson "estimated that the hospital had spent $13 million on so-called charity care in the fiscal year that ended on June 30. In addition, she said, the hospital faced a $16 million bill for state-ordered earthquake retrofitting and could not afford it." The paper went on to report that "Since 1990, 70 hospital emergency rooms and trauma centers have closed in California, a state whose emergency and trauma system is overwhelmed and under-financed, health officials say" (Madigan 2004). It is impossible for us to know the extent to which the prospective costs of complying with SB 1953 were responsible for the hospital closures from 1995 to 2000 and in the following years. Each of the hospitals that closed appears to have been in financial difficulty before the law came into effect. It is reasonable to conclude, however, that the looming costs of compliance affected the decision to close.

In the case of closed emergency rooms in hospitals, however, it is much more likely that they were closed in response to massive financial losses stemming from providing emergency room services. These losses are attributed to the legal requirement for hospitals to treat emergency room patients regardless of their ability to pay. For many lower income persons without healthcare insurance, the emergency room has become the replacement for the family doctor.

5.2.3 Special Challenges for Local Governments

Hospitals owned by counties found themselves in a particularly difficult position. Many of California's general purpose local governments were themselves in desperate financial straits in the 1990s. Their ability to raise taxes to pay for upgrading or replacing hospital facilities and other kinds of infrastructure was severely limited. The State's economy was suffering from the market collapse of sectors of the economy concentrated in California, and Proposition 13 limited the ability of local government to increase revenues from *ad valorem* property taxes. The State government, in an effort to trim its own deficits, continued to cut back on sharing tax revenues with local governments. All states, including California, responded to federal cuts to states for domestic programs by pushing the responsibility for financing onto local governments to the extent possible. Hospital administrators could expect little help from city councils and county boards because healthcare investment decisions were often made by political bodies with little knowledge of healthcare dynamics, because they had different agendas and different constituents, and because they faced intense competition for money from an inadequate purse.

Not only were the State government and general purpose local governments in poor financial shape, but the government-owned hospitals were suffering the same upheavals as not-for-profit and investor-owned hospitals. Like private hospitals, California's local government hospitals faced escalating costs of providing healthcare, reductions in Medicare reimbursements for services rendered, and a growing role of third party payers who bargained for lower fees. Hospitals owned by local governments were generally not in a position to aggressively pursue some of the strategies that were employed successfully by privately-owned organizations to increase their efficiency They were not, for example, in a position to merge with facilities in other communities and other states in an attempt to generate scalar economies.

Administrators of hospitals owned by local governments found themselves caught between a rock and a hard place. They could hardly refuse to comply with SB 1953, at least minimally, even though they had serious financial problems, because so much could be made of the failure to comply by political opponents if the administration did not "make the hospital safe from the threat of collapse." Some hospital administrators decided they had to do something – anything – to comply in the short run, even if doing that something would mean eventually spending a lot more money. To paraphrase one county hospital administrator we interviewed, "We'll cut open the walls and strengthen the column, then close up the hole. If we find pipes in there that are so badly rusted we expect them to break in a matter of weeks, we'll still close up the hole. We simply don't have enough money to fix even obvious problems while we're in there. It's inefficient and stupid, but we don't have a choice."

More than a few local government hospital administrators understood that there was no way they could raise sufficient funds to retrofit their hospitals before 2008 without a major external influx of cash. Few saw how they could arrange for such an influx. Logical, long-term decision making might compel a different approach to addressing seismic issues, one that would take into account the need to modernize facilities and fix any number of issues, but the resources needed to accomplish this were simply not available to most administrators.

In the face of what were perceived as almost intractable challenges, several hospitals owned by special districts created for the express purpose of operating a hospital decided to close. The South Bay Medical Center in Redondo Beach (Los Angeles area) for example, closed in 1998 when Tenet withdrew from a contract to operate the facility for the Beach Cities Hospital District. The Stanislaus County Board of Supervisors closed its hospital facility in 1997 and transferred its patients to a privately owned hospital. The Bloss Memorial District Hospital closed in 1998 and the Lindsay District Hospital closed in 2000.

The story was not, however, completely bleak. Local officials in the City-County of San Francisco saw SB 1953 as a signal that it was time to replace the aging San Francisco General Hospital with a new hospital complex that would meet current seismic standards. In 2008, 84% of voters passed a proposition to finance the new facility with $887.4 million in general obligation municipal bonds. The underlying message to the voters had been that the hospital was required to rebuild in order to meet state seismic standards. According to the San Francisco Department of Public Health, the facility is San Francisco's only trauma center, treats about 100,000 people each year, receives approximately one-third of the city's ambulances and provides 20% of the city's inpatient care (San Francisco Department of Public Health 2010).

A bond referendum for a new hospital also worked in a community located in the Tehachapi Mountains between Bakersfield and Mojave in Kern County, California. The community has a small permanent population, but a large seasonal tourist population. In 2009, Alan Burgess, the Tehachapi Valley Healthcare District CEO, was happy to announce that a $50 million bond that would help pay for the construction of a new hospital passed with about 69% of the vote. A two-thirds affirmative vote was required. Voters had been told that a state mandate would require Tehachapi's current hospital to "shut its doors on January 1, 2013 because it does not meet current seismic standards." Burgess said the new 25-bed critical access facility would meet those standards. The bonds supplemented $15 million in bonds approved in 2004. Donations were expected to provide another half million dollars (Tehachapi 2009).

5.3 First Things First: Seeking Solvency

As indicated above, the primary obstacle to healthcare organizations complying with the retrofit, replace, or change use provisions of SB 1953 was that most of them did not have sufficient resources. Unfortunately, based on our interviews with OSHPD officials, at least a few of those officials were convinced that the healthcare organizations did, in fact, have sufficient financial resources to comply with the regulations, but were simply reluctant to comply. This belief contributed, we think, to a developing adversarial relationship between the regulated and the regulators.

Even as SB 1953 was being developed and enacted, most California hospitals were already focused on and working hard to adapt to the financial upheavals in healthcare. The primary strategy employed by hospital owners to gain solvency in the new milieu was to implement greater efficiencies in conducting their healthcare business. Many sought to create a bigger financial flywheel to level out revenues and expenses by merging with other hospitals. While mergers and restructuring became commonplace, they were not the only adaptive strategies employed. While many hospital organizations attempted to align themselves with a financially stronger organization, others chose to focus on developing a market niche to implement corporate structural changes. In some cases, that meant dividing the original corporation into several corporations as a way to separate those activities with positive cash flows from those with negative cash flows. By having one or more of the separate organizational entities focus on serving the poor and uninsured, individual entities could qualify for serving a "disproportionate share" of those unable to pay and, thus, obtain higher reimbursements from medical assistance programs.

Just as in any other organization, hospital administrators have to set priorities. In the case of SB 1953, there would be no retrofit or replacement at a facility unless the organization achieved solvency in the face of the contextual changes they were experiencing in the late 1990s. In most cases, the decision was to temporarily postpone dealing with the expensive looming requirements of SB 1953 and focus first on achieving solvency. Over and over, hospital administrators told us "No margin, no mission." Thus, their motto became "First things first." Unless they were able to develop a successful strategy for long-term financial viability, they saw no way of complying with the SB 1953 mandates.

5.4 Opting for Replacement Rather Than Retrofit

As hospital owners and managers began to identify and assess their options for compliance, retrofitting existing facilities often became less attractive than replacing those old buildings. Hospital owners understood that retrofitting old buildings to comply with SB 1953 would add to a hospital's fixed costs without providing any significant opportunity to recover those costs.

There were, of course, the normal problems associated with retrofitting any facility. "As-built" drawings of facilities rarely conform entirely to what was actually built or installed. Hidden problems are exposed as walls are opened. Logistic concerns became extremely important to many hospital managers. Cutting open walls and ceilings to make structural and nonstructural changes posed considerable problems. The work would require shuffling patients and activities from place to place around the building while, at the same time, addressing issues arising from possible contamination of patients and staff from dust, bacteria, and viruses loosed by construction. Even non-structural retrofit generated by-product concerns. Our discussions with engineers involved in implementing the regulations indicated that improving some nonstructural elements of individual hospitals also required structural changes and often meant significant disruption of hospital operations. Several hospital administrators we talked with estimated the costs associated with the logistics required to do the retrofits (e.g., disrupting hospital operations, moving patients and activities, building sound and dust barriers, etc.) could be on the order of 60% of the structural and nonstructural work itself. These additional (indirect) costs would increase the costs of compliance far in excess of RAND's estimates of construction and equipment (direct) costs.

Outside the buildings, other logistic problems emerged. Land surrounding most hospital facilities and campuses was not readily available, particularly in urban centers, and it was expensive. If a building had to be replaced, where would the new one be built? Would the perfectly good parking lot or ramp be sacrificed and then be rebuilt on the site of the demolished structure or structures? Managers asked themselves how they could continue operations while building new or undergoing massive structural changes.

For some hospital organizations, retrofit costs represented dollars spent to add a couple of years to the life to an already inadequate building. As hospital administrators examined the option of retrofitting old hospitals or building new, it became clear to many that upgrading outmoded buildings did not make business sense (Jones 2004; Rundle 2004). Some concluded that the dollar cost of retrofitting their facilities could approach more than half the cost of simply building a new building, especially when one considered non-construction logistical costs. This prompted them to consider more seriously the option of rebuilding. In this context, hospital owners were faced with a new decision. Should they skip the retrofit step all together and simply build a new building now? Building new seemed to make economic sense. After all, buildings built before 1973 are usually inefficient in terms of today's medical practice, and require quite a bit of maintenance compared with new buildings. Retrofitting while caring for patients in the same building is, at best, extremely difficult, and a significant proportion of the nonconforming building was functionally obsolete.

While some hospitals closed due, at least in part, to the costs imposed by SB 1953, and while some pondered how to finance and manage retrofit activities, others sought to engage in building programs. Hospitals that were able to survive the financial consequences of changes in the healthcare industry had to become even more competitive to survive. They concluded that new buildings were needed that were congruent with modern medical practice, that incorporated new technologies, and that reduced the need for scarce and expensive medical staff. Those with the financial wherewithal to do so moved in that direction.

"We don't want to just go out and build new versions of old hospitals," said Tony Wagner, executive administrator for hospitals at the San Francisco Department of Public Health. "We should rethink how we are providing care" (Russell 2003).

5.5 The Quest for Legislative Relief

One might argue that the cost of replacing the existing hospital beds in buildings classified as SPC-1 should be a non-issue. After all, by 2008, the newest of these facilities would be 35 years old. Together, they would have a mean age of almost half a century (Meade et al. 2002, p. 12). If the organizations had depreciated the buildings over their assumed lifetime and funded that depreciation, then the fund for depreciation should be able to pay for much of the mandated upgrading. This argument, however, fails to recognize the complexity and the reality of the situation. First, many of the buildings were not built at a single time: many were modified and added to over the years. New wings and other additions were added to what today are considered non-compliant buildings. Second, few organizations actually fund depreciation. Governments and not-for-profit organizations, for the most part, do not.

The governments and not-for-profits that borrow to build and service the bonds over time have a reasonable rationale for not funding depreciation. The argument for paying through borrowing is that the beneficiaries of the service should pay for it; adding debt service to other operating costs when calculating user fees helps to ensure that those who benefit from the facility pay for it. A similar argument could be made for depreciation, except that, if the organization is simultaneously servicing debt incurred to build the facility and funding depreciation, then current users would pay twice.

Most hospitals had few reserves and many had no means for raising or borrowing the large amount of money that would be needed to help them achieve compliance. As many as 85% of the hospitals were operating at a loss. Even if they could somehow borrow the money needed for the remediation or replacement, the debt service would raise their cost curves even higher than the reimbursements they were receiving from the HMOs, Medicare, and other programs. Further, at least in the mind of the hospital owners and operators, the increased costs associated with working toward compliance afforded no means for helping them to remain solvent, much less recapture the investment.

The original framers of the SB 1953 policy had foreseen the need for financial assistance to hospitals. They had included a proposal in their plan for the state government to help hospitals with the costs. That part of the proposed policy ended up "on the cutting room floor" when the legislation was enacted. The State of California was already well into a perennial financial crisis. The legislature simply would not help the hospitals; doing so was out of the question.

A few hospitals were able to fund retrofit or replace old facilities from reserves, borrowing, charitable donations, bond issues, or current income. However, hundreds of hospital owners found themselves in a difficult, perhaps intractable situation. Replacing the hospital typically made the most sense from a long term economic and financial perspective. Retrofitting the old hospital was less expensive, but still carried a heavy price. Even if the hospital could find the resources to complete the retrofit work by 2008, the facility would have to be replaced by 2030.

Besides the financial questions, most administrators with whom we spoke indicated that more pressing concerns kept the possible effects of possible earthquakes on the back burner and off the current agenda. As we talked with them individually, it became clear that most of them thought it was unlikely that an earthquake would cause significant damage or threaten life safety at their location and in their buildings within the foreseeable future. Thus, many believed that they were being asked to spend money to reduce the adverse consequences of an extremely unlikely event. As one healthcare executive told us, "Money spent on seismic 'fixes' to our facilities is money that could be better spent actually delivering healthcare to people who need it."

For these hospitals, the most attractive option available was to seek legislative relief from what they perceived as a tight schedule for compliance or in the form of financial assistance. Seeking legislative relief from regulations they perceive as onerous or costly is a strategy that regulated parties often employ. It was a central element of the strategies employed by many hospital owners in response to SB 1953. Most, but not all, not-for-profit hospital owners and operators appeared from our discussions with them to be willing to comply if it were financially feasible. At least some healthcare organizations hoped to stretch out the time line for compliance and to get some financial assistance from the state or national government.

California's healthcare organizations did not present a wholly united front in their appeal for legislative relief. The positions of hospital owners varied, depending on their individual circumstances. Working both independently and through the California Healthcare Association, many healthcare organizations sought to have the implementation timetable deferred. Others wanted to get financial support from State government. Hospital owners who saw SB 1953 as advantageous to their gaining market share or other advantages provided lukewarm support or none at all in these efforts. Some hospitals were bitterly opposed to the legislation and wanted it repealed. These were typically healthcare organizations with only one or two facilities whose owners saw themselves faced with intractable financial and logistic problems and organizations with buildings they believed to be relatively safe from earthquakes despite their SPC-1 rating. Because individual healthcare organizations had different agendas and objectives, they were unable to agree on a unified legislative position.

In addition, the hospital seismic safety issue had become politicized. The union representing most hospital workers (Service Employees International Union or SEIU) became involved in considerations of the policy, framing it as a "safety in the workplace" issue and opposing the efforts of healthcare organizations to stretch out the compliance timeline. Without a clear, reasonable, and workable proposal backed with near unanimity by the healthcare organizations and supported by the unions, the legislature showed little interest in providing significant relief to healthcare organizations.

There were also institutional reasons for legislative resistance to making major changes in the law. California has legislative term limits. That means that none of the legislators who held office during the quest for legislative relief had been in office when SB 1953 was enacted. Nor would any of those in office when help was sought be there when 2008 rolled around and all hospitals were required to be in compliance. The lobbying organizations, a few legislative staffers, and the officials charged with administering SB 1953 were the only people in Sacramento in whom institutional memory resided, and they each perceived the history through a different lens and from different perspectives. It was, consequently, difficult to drum up much support in the legislature for fixing the problems that healthcare organizations claimed they were facing. Moreover, the State of California's own financial problems were giving state officials serious difficulty. In the final analysis, there were few people in the legislature who might be able to act as a "fixer" in the legislature to address the issues that occurred following adoption and initial implementation of SB 1953.

It was not only healthcare organizations that realized the enormity of the response required by SB 1953. Seismic safety advocates, too, saw the problems associated with implementation. The California Seismic Safety Commission created an *ad hoc* committee to examine compliance with the statute. The committee's creation was precipitated by the Commission's concern that 40% of California's operating hospitals were classified in the highest category of risk of loss of life in the event of an earthquake. The Commission remained steadfast in its call for upgrading those facilities, but, in its November 2001 report, the Commission made several important recommendations (California Seismic Safety Commission 2001). First, the Commission recommended that compliance deadlines be adjusted based on overall reduction of risk to the public. The committee recommended accelerating the 2030 deadline for reconstruction in exchange for extending the 2008 deadline. Second, the Commission urged that deadlines not be extended for individual hospital facilities without evidence of interim progress toward meeting the goals. Third, the Commission recommended that the buildings classified as SPC-1 (those with the least structural seismic resistance) be prioritized for repair or replacement in terms of the level of risk they presented. That is, the Commission suggested that subcategories be developed based on the level of earthquake hazard to which each individual building was likely to be subjected and the vulnerability of the building. Fourth, the Commission recommended that OSHPD invest in applied earthquake research that could make hospital retrofits safer. Fifth, the Commission recommended that hospital owners be encouraged to construct new buildings rather than retrofit older buildings.

The California Seismic Safety Commission made three important additional recommendations concerning State financial assistance for the required improvements. The first of these recommendations was that OSHPD consider the importance of regional hospital coverage when allocating financial assistance for facilities. The second was that the State should provide financial assistance to healthcare organizations based on their individual demonstrated need. The final recommendation was that the State should consider developing incentives other than direct financial assistance for hospitals not eligible for public financing, including accelerated depreciation and funding priorities for federal assistance from organizations like FEMA.

Despite the fact that California healthcare organizations did not have a unified position on what relief, if any, the legislature should provide, and despite the absence of legislators who had created and voted for SB 1953 and the absence of a committed legislative "fixer," considerable activity on SB 1953 took place during the 2000 and 2001 sessions of the California legislature.

SB 1801, introduced by Senator Jackie Speier, became law in the fall of 2000. The original legislation enabled OSHPD to provide a series of 1 year extensions to hospitals for complying with the SB 1953 timetable from 2008 to 2013 under a loss of medical services provision. SB 1801 was intended to provide additional means for hospitals to obtain extensions, but it was written such that only two hospital facilities obtained extensions to 2013 by virtue of SB 1801 (Carlisle and Coleman 2010, p. 13).

SB 2006, introduced by Senator Tim Leslie, recognized the variation in seismicity among areas in the State and provided an exemption for hospital facilities in California's Seismic Zone 3, a zone associated with lower probabilities of severe earthquakes, from certain nonstructural requirement deadlines if the buildings met existing 2002 nonstructural requirements and if hospital owners submitted a site specific geological analysis approved by both OSHPD and the California Division of Mines and Geology (now named the California Geological Survey). The law permits OSHPD to grant hospitals an extension delay to the January 1, 2008 seismic compliance deadline until 2030 for nonstructural requirements (NPC-3 Compliance) if the hospital is *located in Seismic Zone 3* (as indicated in the 1995 edition of the California Building Standards Code) and if the owners have met the NPC 2 requirements and associated deadlines (OSHPD 2005) (*emphasis added by authors*). The law applied only to the Central Valley. It might have applied to areas with similar seismic risks, such as San Diego in Zone 4, had the legislation not specified only Zone 3. It, too, was adopted in the fall of 2000. Since none of the major metropolitan areas were in Seismic Zone 3, the hospitals in those areas did not benefit from the Act.

The legislation that was enacted in 2000 and 2001, along with OSHPD's amendments to the regulations implementing SB 1953, resulted in relatively modest modifications to the timeline for implementing the Hospital Facilities Seismic Safety Act of 1983, as amended, but afforded some needed flexibility from the standpoint of the hospitals (Table 5.1).

A review of the OSHPD's *Summary of Requests for Extensions to Seismic Safety Deadlines* (Office of Statewide Health Planning and Development 2009a) suggests that the overwhelming number of extension requests were classified in the diminished capacity category. Likewise, nearly all requests appear to have been approved.

As of January, 2009, 394 hospitals had applied for extensions to comply with SB 1953 deadlines under the diminished capacity provisions included in the original law. Another 11 hospitals had applied for extensions under the provisions in SB 1801 and 12 had applied for extensions under SB 2006. Table 5.2 shows the number of requests

Table 5.1 Legislation introduced in 2000 and 2001 to provide relief for Healthcare Organizations to comply with SB 1953

Year	Action	Disposition
2000	SB 1801 permits specified, contiguous hospital buildings a 5-year extension of the 2008 deadline if the hospital agrees that the designated services shall be provided by moving into an existing conforming building; relocating to a new building, or retrofitting the existing building that meets the higher year 2030 standards.	Became law in Fall 2000
2000	SB 1886 would require hospitals to submit cost data for compliance to a third party named by OSHPD.	Vetoed
2000	SB 2006 postpones compliance until 2030 for hospital facilities in central and northern California (Seismic Zone 3) from the year 2008 nonstructural bracing requirements if the facilities meet existing 2002 nonstructural requirements and the owners submit a geological analysis.	Became law in Fall 2000
2000	AB 2194 would create a statewide liaison office of hospital seismic safety issues and require hospitals to submit compliance plans for use of temporary facilities.	Became law in Fall 2000
2000	AB 2902 would make a technical correction to SB 1953 to remove sunset on entire Act.	Became law in Fall 2000
2001	AB 1156 would establish a Safe Hospitals Bond Act of 2002.	Died
2001	AB 842 would grant 5-year extension to 2008 for hospitals with at least one building meeting standards.	Died
2001	SB 928 would provide financial assistance to hospitals to comply.	Died
2001	AB 656 would provide relief for Alameda County Hospital to meet 2002 requirements; in process, but can't finish; OSPHD had not issued permit for the work.	Became law in Fall 2001
2001	AB 832 would make all regulatory submissions to California Building Standards Commission by OSHPD emergency regulations, thus speeding the change process.	Became law in Fall 2001
2001	AB 1156 Safe Hospitals Bond Acts.	Died

Source: Developed by the authors from information contained in the State of California Legislative Archives

Table 5.2 Status of applications to OSHPD for SB 1953 extensions as of May 2005

Action taken	Diminished capacity	%, distribution	SB 1801	%, distribution	SB 2006	%, distribution
Pending	1	0.5	1	9.1	1	8.3
Denied	2	0.3	7	63.6	1	8.3
Approved	391	99.2	2	27.3	10	83.3
Total	394	100.0	10	100.0	12	100.0

Source: California Office of Statewide Health Planning, *Summary of Requests for Extensions to Seismic Safety Deadlines*, January 28, 2009

and actions taken. Of these, 94.7% cited "diminished capacity." That is, they maintained that complying with SB 1953 would result in an interruption of healthcare services provided by general acute care hospitals within their service area. Diminished capacity provides for extensions in 1-year increments for up to 5 years beyond January 1, 2008. Only two of the hospitals claiming diminished capacity were denied extensions and one application was pending as of January 2009.

Hospitals were also able to request extensions to compliance deadlines if they agreed that on or before January 1, 2013, they would relocate into a new building or retrofit a noncomplying building to meet designated seismic performance standards. Ten hospitals applied under this provision (SB 1801). Six were denied and only two approved.

The legislature was generally sympathetic to requests to provide relief in the form of stretched timelines, but was steadfastly opposed to providing financial assistance to hospital organizations, despite their claims of financial and logistic constraints. All legislative attempts to provide financial assistance to hospitals in 2000 and 2001 died in the legislature. The California legislature was simply not going to provide financial assistance to support SB 1953 implementation. This was understandable in the context of the State of California's dire fiscal condition. Virtually all the states in the Union were suffering the fiscal effects of the recession, federal devolution of costs to the states, and massive financial pressure from healthcare entitlement programs, particularly for the elderly, but California appeared to be suffering more than most (Shattuck Hammond 2001). Bills submitted to the California legislature seeking support for helping to implement SB 1953 with financial assistance to hospitals for rebuilding and retrofit got nowhere.

Given the unwillingness of the State of California to provide financial assistance to hospitals, hospital owners sought financial assistance from the Federal government through the California Congressional delegation. Senator Dianne Feinstein introduced legislation in 2001 for Federal support, but the bill was derailed following the September 11 terrorist attacks (Sticker 2004). Congressman Jerry Lewis of Orange County, California introduced a similar bill (H.R. 1669) in the House, but it did not go further.

5.6 The Voters Put Some of the Cost Burden onto the State's Shoulders

Despite the legislative resistance demonstrated in the first half of the decade, the State did finally find itself shouldering some of the financial burden of bringing acute care, in-patient facilities into compliance. It was not, however, because the legislature changed its mind about financing enhanced hospital seismic safety. California permits "initiative, referendum, and recall" at both the state and local level. Citizens, on their own initiative, can place binding propositions on ballots, providing they get a sufficient number of signatures.

Assembly member Dion Louise Aroner, representing communities in the East Bay area of San Francisco Bay, had introduced a bill on February 23, 2001 calling for a "Safe Hospitals Bond Act of 2002." If adopted, it would authorize the issuance of an unspecified amount of bonds "for construction, replacement, renovation, and retrofit of currently licensed health facilities that are subject to, and for purposes of meeting the requirements of, the Alfred E. Alquist Hospital Facilities Seismic Safety Act." The bill would provide for submitting the bond act to the voters at the March 5, 2002, statewide primary election. It died in the legislature.

Those interested in having the State shoulder some of the financial burden of enhancing seismic safety in hospitals did not give up easily. They employed the initiative process to further their goal. In 2004, Proposition 61, known as the Children's Hospital Bond Act of 2004, was placed on the ballot. It was enacted with more than 58% of those casting a ballot voting in favor of authorizing $750 million in general obligation bonds to provide funding for construction, expansion, remodeling, renovating, furnishing, and equipping hospitals that focus on children. One-fifth of the money was ear-marked for specified University of California hospitals and 80% was targeted for general acute care hospitals that focus on children with illnesses such as leukemia, heart defects, and so forth.

A second proposition, known as Proposition 3, was on the ballot in 2008. It was nearly identical to the 2004 proposition, except that it called for a $980 million dollar bond issue. It, too, passed and became law. Today, this amount would cover the costs of only one or two replacement hospitals. Nonetheless, through the California process known as initiative and referendum, the State of California found itself using its full faith and credit borrowing power to finance about $1.7 billion of hospital construction aimed, to a considerable extent, on replacing hospitals that had been classified at SPC-1.

Both Proposition 61 and Proposition 3 bore a striking resemblance to Assemblywoman Aroner's 2001 bill that died in the legislature. The names were different. The failed bill was entitled the "Safe Hospitals Bond Act of 2002." The successful propositions were entitled the "Children's Hospital Bond Act of 2004" and the "Children's Hospital Bond Act of 2006." Despite the name changes, the bonds would help finance compliance with SB 1953.

5.7 OSHPD'S Construction Loan Insurance Program

Since 1972, a Division of OSHPD has been insuring loans to healthcare facilities at no cost to the State of California. Cal-Mortgage administers the California Health Facility Construction Loan Insurance Program (Office of Statewide Health Planning and Development 2009b). The program insures loans to non-profit healthcare facilities with the full faith and credit of the State, helping the owners of those facilities obtain loans at the same or lower rates than the State of California. Since the program was initiated, it has insured more than $6 billion in loans to more than 500 healthcare facilities.

Cal-Mortgage provides an excellent opportunity for not-for-profit healthcare organizations to obtain loans, provided they are able to demonstrate a capacity to service the debt. The challenge, of course, is for the hospital to convince themselves and lenders that they will be able to service the debt. As it turns out, Cal-Mortgage has outstanding loan guarantees to only nine general acute care hospitals with a total loan balance in 2009 of $718,569,000. Loans to six of the nine are classed as having no problems or only minor problems. Default is anticipated in two loans and another has "moderate" problems. In 2009, Cal-Mortgage was insuring about 115 loans to other kinds of healthcare facilities, including day care facilities for developmentally disabled adults, continuing care retirement facilities, skill nursing facilities, mental health clinics, and primary care clinics, among others. Thus, while Cal-Mortgage help is available for relatively low interest loan guarantees, few hospitals are affording themselves of OSHPD's services in that area, perhaps because they do not believe that borrowing, even at low interest, is a feasible alternative for them.

5.8 OSHPD Seeks Relief

Not all the legislative relief was sought by the hospitals. OSHPD also sought relief. It was faced with enormous workloads as a consequence of the large number of facility plans to be evaluated, and because it was aware of the difficulties many hospitals were encountering. Normally, it takes about 18 months to make changes to administrative regulations in California. Emergency changes to administrative regulations, however, can be approved much more quickly. Understanding the need to respond quickly to problems that emerged as SB 1953 implementation proceeded, OSHPD, with others, sought to have changes to SB 1953s administrative regulations classified as emergency changes. The legislature provided OSHPD with welcome relief in 2001 by enacting a bill that would make all regulatory submissions to California Building Standards Commission by OSHPD emergency regulations, thus speeding the change process. The bill was introduced in February 2001 (AB 832) and was supported by both the Seismic Safety Commission and the California Hospital Association. It passed both houses and was signed into law in September of that same year.

OSHPD administrators also tried to get an exception to a hiring freeze imposed on State agencies because of the State's financial problems. OSHPD was understaffed relative to the massive workload associated with SB 1953. Despite the fact that the hospital organizations were paying fees that covered the administrative costs of processing their plans and applications and, even though no tax revenues would be used for salaries and other expenses, OSHPD was unsuccessful in its attempts to gain relief from the hiring freeze. As a result, the time required for the program administrators to reply to hospital owners and operators became a hindrance to both the hospitals and the agency itself.

5.9 Seismic Safety: One Consideration Among Many in the Hospital Business Plan

One consequence of the emphasis on "first things first" resulted in many healthcare organizations transforming themselves from organizations that focused mainly on delivering healthcare services into businesses that continued to deliver healthcare services while also paying serious attention to costs, product mix, marketing, and strategic planning. The change was forced on them by the dynamic context within which they found themselves. Survival required successful adaptation. Successful adaptation required change. By 2004, a significant proportion of California's investor-owned hospitals had begun to turn a profit, and, in the case of not-for-profit hospitals, an operating surplus. The proportion of hospitals with net operating losses began to shrink as adaptors survived and non-adaptors closed their doors.

The picture at mid-decade was not entirely rosy for hospitals. California hospitals in the 75th percentile of financial performance in 2005 received 63% of their revenue from private payers. Those in the 25th percentile received only 35% of their revenue from those sources and 63% from Medicare and Medi-Cal, California's healthcare support for low income and indigent persons While the providers of the data on which the conclusions are drawn indicate the data are subject to some caveats, it appears that over half California's hospitals had bond ratings below investment grade, ranging from bbb to Junk (Price Waterhouse Coopers June 2007).

As some healthcare organizations began to benefit financially from their transformation, they began to look at complying with SB 1953 within a strategic business context. These administrators did not look at the problem as a structural problem. They saw it in terms of a business decision to be made in terms of corporate goals and strategies for achieving those goals. The question posed was no longer "should we retrofit and, if so, how?" or "should we rebuild?" Rather, the choices to of how to comply with SB 1953 and how to mitigate earthquake risks were always weighed in a strategic context along with other priorities. The healthcare and organizational contexts were always dynamic and infused with great uncertainty about the near future, much less the longer term. Only rarely was the corporate decision driven by the availability of an engineering solution. In fact, the availability of one engineering solution often prompted decision makers to ask technical staff and consultants for more and different engineering solutions, so that any final decisions reflected more than the quickest or most obvious fix. The corporate decision was made more difficult when they sought opinions about what it would take to retrofit their structures from more than one structural engineer and received answers with strikingly different cost estimates. The cost estimates may have assumed vastly different scopes. For example, the addition of ADA (Americans with Disabilities Act) upgrades can add 20% to construction costs.

Based on our discussions with healthcare executives and others involved in the decision making process, it seems to us that healthcare organizations approached the question of whether to retrofit, rebuild, or close iteratively, cycling back and forth through an amalgam of identified problems, possible solutions, relevant players, and likely costs and consequences. Thus, the conversation might begin with "Should we retrofit the structure?" From there, questions might include, "If not, what could we do with the building? Sell it or perhaps change its use to something other than acute care?" "Should we even keep the building? Perhaps we should replace it." "Well, should we even keep that facility open? Can it generate enough revenue to cover the costs? Does it fit into our mission? Is it the right location?" And, even, "Can we afford to stay in business, or should we fold?"

We think that individual hospitals and healthcare organizations have always known that they needed to be competitive to survive; we also think that meeting the demands of the operating environment of the 1990s meant that hospital owners and managers found that the old ways of being competitive were not working in the new context. They needed to learn new lessons in what it meant to be competitive and avoid organizational entropy in the new context. Some hospitals did not or could not adapt, and did not survive. Other hospitals learned how to adapt, and some even thrived in the new financial environment. They became more sophisticated and learned how to gain access to new resources.

We also think that competitive strategies (e.g., low cost, differentiation, focus) contributed to the demand for new buildings. High labor costs and shortages of skilled personnel demanded new labor-saving approaches, and new healthcare technologies and methods demanded new kinds of space. At the same time, we think that healthcare organizations that had hoped that SB 1953 was going to go away finally concluded that it was not. There might have been some options for delaying compliance, but, in general, the requirement for stronger and safer acute care hospital buildings remained in force. Finally, we think that the goals of SB 1953 were furthered when it became financially advantageous for healthcare organizations to replace old, outmoded buildings with new ones rather than attempt to retrofit. Though organizations might publicly point to SB 1953 as a "trigger" or "compelling force" behind their decision to rebuild, in fact it was other considerations that tilted their decision toward a new facility (e.g., desire to upgrade their buildings in line with modern medical practice, in order to attract certain doctors and patients).

Traditionally, capital improvements for investor-owned buildings are financed through a combination of operating cash flow, corporate reserves, new investor equity, and debt. Local government typically builds hospitals by borrowing money with either general obligation or revenue bonds. Not-for-profit organizations use a combination of capital fund-raising from philanthropists and borrowing. Investor-owned firms finance from the sale of shares, equity, and borrowing. In addition, hospitals often benefit from governmental subsidies for construction. As we saw earlier in this chapter, borrowing has not been an option for most healthcare organizations.

In the end, the need to generate a profit or surplus is a day-to-day concern for hospital owners, whereas the need to remain operational after an earthquake is not, except for organizations like Kaiser Permanente, which has already collected its premiums and is required to provide care to its members. That is a very different business model from most hospital providers. Since the day-to-day tends to be more salient than the rare but potentially ruinous event, and since the issues on the front burner are more salient and tend to be addressed first, it should come as no surprise that the choice of how to comply with SB 1953 might flow more from the desire to generate revenue than from the desire to protect against the virtual certainty of experiencing a significant earthquake, but the low probability that it will be anytime soon. Given their concerns about continued viability and their lack of financial resources, many hospital owners continued with their efforts to buy time beyond 2008 in hopes that they could devise more and better options.

References

California Seismic Safety Commission (2001) Seismic Safety Commission findings and recommendations on hospital seismic safety, November

Carlisle DM, Coleman PA (2010) California senate health committee hearing on hospital seismic safety, 3 Mar 2010. Testimony by the Office of Statewide Health Planning and Development (OSHPD)

Catholic Health World (2003) CHW facilities seek more time for seismic retrofit, 5 Nov 2003

Jones WJ (2004) Renewal by earthquake: designing 21st century hospitals in response to California's seismic safety legislation. New Century HealthCare Institute, Oakland

Kaiser Permanente (2010) http://xnet.kp.org/newscenter/aboutkp/historyofkp.html

Madigan N (2004) Los Angeles emergency care crisis deepens. The New York Times, 21 Aug 2004

Meade C, Kulick J, Hillestad R (2002) Estimating the compliance costs for California SB 1953. California HealthCare Foundation, Oakland

Nicholas C. Petris Center (2001) California's closed hospitals, 1995–2000. Nicholas C. Petris Center on health care markets and consumer welfare, April. University of California, Berkeley, School of Public Health, Berkeley

Office of Statewide Health Planning and Development (2009a) Summary of requests for extensions to seismic safety deadlines, 28 January. California Office of Statewide Health Planning and Development, Facilities Development Division, Sacramento

Office of Statewide Health Planning and Development (2009b) Cal-Mortgage loan insurance program. Office of Statewide Health Planning and Development, Cal-Mortgage Loan Insurance Division, Sacramento

Price Waterhouse Coopers (2007) Financial health of California hospitals. California Healthcare Association, Sacramento, June

Rundle RL (2004) Career FYI: top trends affecting U.S. hospitals. Wall Str J Online. www.careerjournal.com/salaryhiring/industries/health/20041209-rundle.html

Russell S (2003) Hospital building boom ahead: earthquake safety forcing private, public medical centers to rebuild or retrofit. San Francisco Chronicle, June 8. Retrieved 2 June 2005 from: http://www.sfgate.com/cgi-bin/article.cgi?file=/c/a/2003/06/08/MN3240.DTL

San Francisco Department of Public Health (2010) Rebuild SF General Hospital. (http://www.sfdph.org/dph/rebuildSFGH)

Shattuck Hammond Partners (2001) The financial health of California hospitals. Shattuck Hammond Partners, San Francisco, July

Sticker M (2004) Earthquake codes shake California hospitals to the core, health care insider, 5 Mar 2004

Tehachapi News (2009). http://www.tehachapinews.com/content/voters-approve-hospital-bond

University of California-Davis (2010) Health system, facilities design and construction update http://www.ucmdc.ucdavis.edu/construction/siteimpacts/sb1953.html. Last accessed 18 Aug 2011

Vogt K (2004) Tenet announces major sell-off. American Medical News, 16 Feb 2004

Chapter 6
Implementation: Circa 2005 Through 2010

6.1 Prognosis at Mid-Decade

During 2006, RAND analysts updated their 2002 cost estimates for achieving compliance with SB 1953 and identified factors they believed to be significant challenges to implementing the program (Meade and Kulick 2007). Meade and Kulick (2007) concluded what many participants in the process already knew. The pace of SB 1953 compliance was slow during the first half of the decade. Meade and Kulick assessed data on historical rates of construction and permit filings with OSHPD and concluded that compliance would likely not meet the deadlines imposed. In fact, they concluded that about half the SPC-1buildings would not meet the 2008–2013 compliance deadlines and that many might not comply with the final 2030 deadline.

Compliance lagged because the majority of California hospitals had serious financial problems from enactment in 1994 well into the first decade of the new century and the costs of complying with SB 1953 continued to rise at a rapid rate. Meade and Kulick updated their estimated costs of compliance with SB 1953 to reflect the experience during the 5 years since their 2002 estimates.

> (C)ost scenarios (were made) accounting for trade-offs in inflation rates, construction rates, and the sizing of new facilities. With plausible parameters for these factors, the scenarios indicate that the total construction could cost \$45 billion to \$110 billion, in 2006 dollars. This estimate does not account for the cost of financing, which could increase the total by as much as a factor of two (Meade and Kulick 2007).

Meade and Kulick's (2007) estimated increases in costs were substantial, particularly since the estimate did not include the costs of rebuilding SPC-2 buildings which must be replaced by 2030.

The estimated costs of compliance with SB 1953 had increased from early estimates of about \$14 billion to as high as \$110 billion in a matter of just a decade. Perhaps one significant reason for the increased cost estimates were that the earliest estimates might be characterized more as gucsses than as rigorous cost estimates. Meade and Kulick's estimates were based on methods of estimating aggregate costs

D.J. Alesch et al., *Natural Hazard Mitigation Policy: Implementation, Organizational Choice, and Contextual Dynamics*, Environmental Hazards,
DOI 10.1007/978-94-007-2235-4_6,

that had been developed by RAND over decades. Perhaps more importantly, they were based on better information than that which was available before program adoption and in the first years of implementation. As structural engineers began to address the problems of individual hospital buildings and got feedback from the OSHPD regulators, they developed a better understanding of what would have to be done to achieve compliance and, as a consequence, a better understanding of the costs. In the first few years of working on SB 1953 compliance, there were some strikingly different estimates by individual engineers of what would be required to retrofit individual facilities and, thus, large variations in cost estimates. There was a steep learning curve that began to result in a narrower, but significantly higher range of estimated cost.

In addition, Meade and Kulick noted changes in hospital design, making them larger and with increased design standards. They attributed a significant share of their increased cost estimate to those changes. Yet another important reason for increased costs was rapid and major inflation in the cost of commodities required for either retrofitting or building new hospital facilities. "For complex buildings such as hospitals, per-foot prices that were $330 per square foot in 2003 have gone up to $550 per square foot in mid-2006" (Greene 2006). Demand for building materials generated in China, India, and by Hurricane Katrina helped to push up the costs of steel, copper, concrete, asphalt, aluminum, and PVC piping dramatically. Copper, for example, increased in price by 87% from mid-2005 to mid-2006.

6.2 Hospital Financial Problems Persist

In 2001, 38% of California's hospitals had negative total margins. That is, income from all sources was less than expenses. By 2007, that proportion decreased to 33%, about a 20% improvement. Only about one-fifth of hospitals owned by not-for-profit organizations experienced total negative margins in 2007, the best ratio among the various types of hospital owners. Of the California hospitals owned by special districts and other governments, 47% and 40%, respectively, experienced overall losses in 2007. In that same year, more than half (55%) of investor-owned hospitals reported that costs exceeded income from all sources.

By 2007, most of the hospitals that survived the first half of the decade had instituted significant changes in an attempt to cope with reductions in reimbursements from insurance companies and public healthcare programs and rapidly rising costs. Just as they were learning how to cope with those challenges, another serious challenge arose. The amount of charity care increased 23% (inflation adjusted dollars) from 2001 to 2007 and, during the same period, bad debts increased by 19% (California Health Care Foundation 2010).

The Emergency Medical Treatment and Active Labor Act of 1985 (EMTALA) obligates hospitals to treat the uninsured but does not pay for that care. The law states that:

> In the case of a hospital that has a hospital emergency department, if any individual comes to the emergency department and a request is made on the individual's behalf for examination or treatment for a medical condition, the hospital must provide for an appropriate

> medical screening examination within the capability of the hospital's emergency department, including ancillary services routinely available to the emergency department, to determine whether or not an emergency medical condition . . . exists . . . If any individual. . . comes to a hospital and the hospital determines that the individual has an emergency medical condition, the hospital must provide either within the staff and facilities available at the hospital, for such further medical examination and such treatment as may be required to stabilize the medical condition, or for transfer of the individual to another medical facility . . .(United States Code 42).

Unprecedented numbers of uninsured and impoverished people began using emergency rooms as their "family physician" following passage of the Act, with the numbers growing exponentially in southern California in the first decade of the twenty-first century. With the dramatic increases in healthcare insurance and growing unemployment and underemployment, many who were once insured were now uninsured. Certainly, the recession that began mid decade and continued at the time of this writing accounts for a significant portion of the increase in unpaid medical services received. Anecdotal evidence suggests, too, that a large proportion of uninsured and low income persons using emergency rooms in southern California is made up of undocumented immigrants. Perhaps because it is viewed as politically incorrect, few, if any, studies have appeared in the scholarly literature concerning the reasons for and the demographic composition of the huge increase in charity care in southern California emergency rooms. Nonetheless, the large and rapid increases in bad debt and charity service have contributed to the ongoing financial problems of California hospitals. The Los Angeles Times reported that 61 California hospitals closed from 1998 to 2007, most of which had emergency rooms in 1998 and which were closed either before the hospital closed or at the same time.

Since 1972, the State of California has provided a self-funded mortgage insurance program to assist healthcare organizations by enabling them to use the State's credit to borrow money for improvements at interest rates lower than they might otherwise be able to obtain in the bond market. Cal-Mortgage, located within OSHPD, administers the program. Loans are insured for a wide range of healthcare facilities, including "hospitals, of any type, skilled nursing facilities, intermediate care facilities, public health centers, clinics and other outpatient facilities, multi-level facilities (which include a residential facility for the elderly operated in conjunction with an intermediate care facility, a skilled nursing facility, or a general acute care hospital), laboratories, community mental health centers, facilities for the treatment of chemical dependency, child day care facilities in conjunction with a health facility, adult day health centers, group homes, facilities for the developmentally disabled or mentally disordered, (and) offices and central service facilities operated in connection with a health facility" (Cal-Mortgage Loan Insurance Program, October 3, 2008).

The Cal-Mortgage loan insurance program, however, has not played a major role in helping to finance general acute care hospitals efforts to comply with SB 1953. As of 2009, the program insured only 19 loans to general acute care hospitals (Table 6.1). Of those 19 loans, eight were reported to have no problems, six had minor problems, one had moderate problems, and two were classified as "default anticipated" (Cal-Mortgage 2010). The fact that Cal-Mortgage insures such a small

Table 6.1 Outstanding Cal-Mortgage loan insurance policies to General Acute Care Hospitals, 2009

Location by city	Number of outstanding loans	Current principal balance	Risk rating
Chico	2	$35,595,000	A: no problems
El Centro	1	$32,800,000	A: no problems
Hayward	2	$42,100,000	B: minor problems
Lodi	2	$152,985,000	A: no problems
Oroville	2	$16,145,000	E: default anticipated
Panorama City	1	$29,890,000	C: moderate problems
Placerville	4	$77,885,000	B: minor problems
Valencia	3	$123,240,000	A: no problems
Victorville	2	$7,928,782	C: moderate problems
Totals	**19**	**$718,568,782**	

Source: Cal-Mortgage loan insurance legislative reports, report 1 – Financial Status of Borrowers, 2009 financial status report

number of loans for general acute care hospitals could be the result of several factors. Hospitals in financial trouble may see no reason to apply for loan insurance because they have concluded that they could not service the debt. Hospitals in good financial condition may be able to obtain better rates on their own because the state's financial problems have been reflected in what it must pay to sell bonds. According to one report, in 2008, California's "general obligation bonds maturing in 2038, with a stated interest rate of 5.25%, traded at 81.9 cents on the dollar to yield about 6.66%, according to the municipal securities rulemaking board. That's 1.57% points more than 3 months ago" (Marois 2008).

6.3 Lagging Implementation Spurs Governmental Adaptations

No one was eager to have OSHPD put in a position where it would have to attempt to remove a hospital's license. Removing the license of a hospital providing critical services to a community would be politically messy and generate issues no one really wanted to contemplate nor with which anyone wanted to deal. Elected state officials could not possibly be comfortable with the prospect of OSHPD revoking the licenses of perhaps 200 acute care hospitals. OSHPD officials would not want to be in a position of being forced to invoke the sanctions called for in the legislation. Hospital owners were not interested in closing their doors and forsaking their missions or with getting into a messy and extended confrontation with OSHPD. Indeed, it was in everyone's interests for the acute care hospitals to be in compliance. Nonetheless, it was clear to almost every observer by mid-decade that many hospital organizations would not be able to comply with the 2008 deadline.

Meade and Kulick noted in their January 2007 report that "in practice, the SB 1953 deadlines have been moved ahead by 17–22 years" (Meade and Kulick 2007, p. 5). The legislative changes between 1998 and 2005 represented a response to heavy lobbying by the regulated parties and an acknowledgement by the State legislature and executive branch that enhancing seismic safety in California's older hospital facilities was considerably more than a technical exercise in retrofitting or replacing those buildings. The problem was a lot more complex, more expensive, more time-consuming, and more political than those who devised the policy had ever envisaged.

In this context, some hospital owners continued their efforts to comply with pending deadlines, some hospitals closed, and others continued to seek ways to comply or to extend the dates for compliance.

6.3.1 SB 1661: An Extension for Facilities with Active Compliance Projects Delayed for Circumstances Beyond Their Control

In 2006, the California legislature enacted Senate Bill 1661 to amend the Health and Safety Code and it was signed into law by the Governor. Introduced by the late Senator David Cox representing the Sacramento area, the bill authorizes OSHPD to grant an additional compliance extension if a hospital is making reasonable progress toward meeting the timeline set forth, but "factors beyond the hospital's control" make it impossible for the hospital to meet the compliance deadline. The hospital applying for the extension is required to meet stringent conditions. First, the hospital building must be under construction at the time of the request for extension and the purpose of the construction must be to meet SB 1953 requirements to use the building as a general acute care hospital building. Second, the hospital building plans had to have been submitted to OSHPD "ready for review" by OSHPD at least 4 years prior to the applicable deadline for the building. Third, the hospital had to have received a building permit for the building at least 2 years before the applicable deadline for the building. Extensions would be granted to 2015 (California State Senate 2006).

The opportunity for obtaining the extension applied to a relatively few hospitals, but it recognized the consequences of the tight compliance schedule, given the complexity of design, time-consuming review and design change processes, and project construction.

6.3.2 SB 306: Recognizing the Constraints of Financial Capacity

Introduced by Senator Denise Ducheny in 2007, SB 306 would authorize hospital owners "who do not have the financial capacity to bring certain buildings into compliance by 2013 to, instead, replace the buildings by January 1, 2020" (California Senate 2007). "The 2020 Seismic Safety Extension allows city or county hospitals or hospitals that meet strict financial hardship criteria to receive a 7 year extension from the 2013 seismic safety deadlines and instead require the hospitals to replace those buildings by 2020" (OSHPD 2009). This law provided those hospitals that qualify another 7 years (12 years beyond the original 2008 deadline) to comply. The *quid pro quo* for the extension would be that they would have to replace their noncompliant facilities 10 years earlier than the date originally stipulated for replacement, in 2020.

Arguments for and against the legislation were similar to those for preceding legislation to alter the compliance deadlines for SB 1953. The California Hospital Association (CHA) said that,

> . . . hospitals are facing extreme challenges in meeting the 2008 and 2013 seismic deadlines. Many will be unable to meet the deadlines because of financial difficulties. For those that have the resources to build or retrofit, other challenges have presented themselves over the past few years, including rising construction costs, review delays, contractor limitations, and necessary plan modifications. This bill provides an extension to hospitals that are working in good faith toward meeting the 2008 and 2013 deadlines. Unless they are provided an extension, these hospitals will be forced to close their existing acute care facility until construction of the new facility was complete, eliminating needed hospital services in many communities (California Legislative Information 2007).

The California Nurses Association has been steadfast in its opposition to legislation that would provide healthcare organizations with relief from the existing deadlines. Just like the testimony for the bill, the Association's opposition to SB 306 followed its traditional arguments.

> Hospitals have known for a very long time that they must comply with the seismic standards by 2008 and 2030; some have complied, over 200 have asked for and received extensions until 2013, and some have done nothing at all. CNA argues that a hospital's failure to plan for future construction needs is no excuse to jeopardize the safety of patients and hospital employees and the bill could encourage some hospitals who have consistently failed to plan for their seismic upgrades to continue to procrastinate (California State Senate Health Committee 2007).

The bill was supported by American Federation of State, County and Municipal Employees, AFL-CIO, the California Hospital Association, the City of San Diego, the Daughters of Charity Health System, the Service Employees International Union, Stanford Hospital, the American Institute of Architects California Council, and the University of California. It was opposed only by the California Nurses Association. The bill passed unanimously in the state Senate and 70 to 2 in the Assembly. When signed into law by Governor Schwarzenegger, in October 2007, the law represented a clear recognition that a significant number of hospitals in the State were unable to comply with the regulations for financial reasons. It is likely that the potential consequences of not granting the extensions appeared to elected officials to be far greater than the consequences of granting the extensions.

6.3.3 A Major Programmatic Adaptation: Using HAZUS to Reclassify Many Buildings from SPC-1 to SPC-2

In enacting SB 1953, seismic safety advocates had inadvertently generated a complex problem of major proportions. There were too many hospitals to rehabilitate or replace, too much money needed, too many healthcare organizations with too little money, too much complexity, and too little time. Rescinding the law was not an option. Some healthcare organizations had already spent millions to comply and dozens of projects were in the works. Moreover, the issue was politicized with interests already raising major objections to every proposal in the state legislature for extensions to the timeline. Moreover, no one wanted to be pointed out as having allowed hospitals "in danger of collapse" to threaten the lives of patients and to be unable to serve the injured in the event of an earthquake. There was no way to turn back the clock. A way out was needed. Since neither the legislative nor executive branches was able to come forth with that way out, it was left to the agency and to seismic safety advocates to find it.

The solution that was ultimately devised and adopted had actually been proposed in 2001by the California Seismic Safety Commission's *ad hoc* committee to examine compliance with the statute. In its November 2001 report, the Commission recommended that compliance deadlines be adjusted based on overall reduction of risk to the public presented by individual structures. Specifically, the committee recommended that the buildings classified as SPC 1 (those with the least structural seismic resistance) be prioritized for repair or replacement in terms of the level of risk they presented. What remained to be done was to find a credible method for prioritizing the buildings and to have the legislature approve doing so.

A long-time seismic safety advocate and well-respected structural engineer, William Holmes, was instrumental in helping to identify and promote a credible method for prioritizing the hospitals so that OSHPD could address "the worst first." Working with OSHPD's John Gillengarten who, at that time, was Deputy Director of the Facility Development Division, Holmes contacted Dr. Charles Kircher who had created HAZUS for the Federal Emergency Management Agency (FEMA) in the mid-1990s. HAZUS (Hazards United States) is a loss estimation methodology that has become the national standard for estimating probable losses from natural hazard events. The model was developed to help public officials prepare for emergency response and community recovery. HAZUS was intended originally to provide aggregate loss estimates. If it were to be useful in prioritizing hospitals for retrofit or replacement, it would have to be modified so that it could be applied to individual structures. Working with staff from a structural engineering firm, Kircher was able to do so and, in September 2008, John Gillengarten, Chris Tokas, and Roy Lobo, all OSHPD staff, presented a paper at the annual convention of the Structural Engineers Association of California (SEAOC) entitled "Reassessment and Reprioritization of SPC-1 Hospital Buildings." It outlined the application of HAZUS to the task of establishing hospital retrofit or replacement priorities (Gillengarten and Tokas 2008).

In the paper, Gillengarten and his colleagues recalled that the procedures employed by OSHPD for the initial classification of hospitals were based on "FEMA 178: NEHRP Handbook for the Seismic Evaluation of Existing Buildings." They continued by writing that, "Since the publication of FEMA 178, significant progress has been made in understanding the seismic performance of buildings, especially in performance based design." They reported that OSHPD proposed using

> . . . the Advanced Engineering Building Module (AEBM) of Hazards U.S. Multi-Hazard (HAZUS-MH), a new state-of-the-art methodology, to reassess the SPC-1 buildings and reprioritize them based on their level of seismic risk. Those SPC-1 buildings that exceed the maximum allowable risk would have to comply with the 2008/2013 deadline.

Buildings that are determined to be at a lower seismic risk will be reclassified to SPC-2 and would have until 2030 to comply with seismic safety requirements (Gillengarten and Tokas 2008).

The expectation was clearly that the HAZUS analysis would provide a more accurate assessment of the potential for building collapse in the event of an earthquake than the methods employed in 2000, the time during which buildings were being evaluated. If the proposal were adopted, Gillengarten and his colleagues said, hospital owners would have a state-of-the-art methodology for potentially having SPC-1 buildings reclassified to SPC-2. Using HAZUS would be voluntary; hospital owners would have the option of requesting a collapse probability assessment.

On October 11, 2009, Governor Arnold Schwarzenegger signed into law SB 499 authorizing the use of HAZUS for establishing retrofit or replacement priorities. The bill had been authored by Senator Denise Ducheny and submitted through the Senate's Health Committee which was chaired at the time by Senator Elaine K. Alquist, the wife of former Senator Alfred E. Alquist. He had championed the original seismic safety legislation, but had been "termed out" by California's term limit law and she had replaced him.

SB 499 made adjustments to the reporting requirements for hospitals. It required that all owners of a general acute care hospital classified as a nonconforming SPC-1 building who requested an extension for compliance beyond January 1, 2008, to file a status and progress report to OSHPD by June 30, 2011 and that OSHPD place that information on its web site within 90 days of receiving the report (California State Senate 2009). More importantly, the legislation authorized OSHPD to use HAZUS "for the purpose of determining the structural performance category of general acute care hospital buildings" (California State Senate Health Committee 2009). The bill authorized OSHPD to promulgate regulations to implement the provision and required OSHPD would submit the regulations to the California Building Standards Commission for approval as emergency regulations.

As of September 2, 2010, 289 hospital buildings had been reclassified from SPC-1 to SPC-2 on the basis of a HAZUS reassessment. This meant that they would not have to be replaced until 2030 instead of 2008 or, if they had other exceptions and extensions, by 2013, or 2015, or 2020. HAZUS was employed because it was said to be an improvement on the best available approach that had been incorporated into the SB 1953 program for classifying the seismic resistance of buildings when the law was enacted in 1994.

One reason, perhaps, that some of the buildings originally classified as SPC-1 were able to be reclassified as SPC-2 buildings, and thus delaying their need to be replaced until 2030, is definitional. The original criterion of "posing a significant risk of collapse and a danger to the public" was a 0.75% chance that the building would fail in the event of specified ground motion. That is, there was a probability of 99.25% that the building would *not* collapse in the event of that ground motion. Under the more sophisticated methodology embraced in the HAZUS analysis, the maximum collapse threshold for any single building was increased to 1.2%, thus changing the probability of not collapsing given the specified ground motion to 98.8%. That is, by almost any measure, a relatively small increase in permissible vulnerability but it enabled the healthcare industry to focus on what one person called "the worst of the worst first." Moreover, the new rules permitted hospitals to make voluntary improvements to buildings so that they could meet the new standards for SPC-2 and thus defer the need for replacement to 2030. One well-respected engineering firm noted how this would benefit one of its clients:

> For an estimated cost of $8 million, this approach will reduce the number of deficiencies and yield a probability of collapse less than 1.2% for both buildings. With a probability of collapse less than 1.2%, both buildings will be able to be reclassified as SPC-2. This gives the hospital another ten years to determine to replace or upgrade to current code by 2030 (Barnard 2010).

6.3.4 Legislative Adjustments Continue into 2010

Shortly after the California Building Safety Commission adopted emergency regulations permitting the use of HAZUS, Senator Ducheny introduced SB 289 which, at the time of this writing, was still active in the legislature. SB 289 has been referred to as a "spot bill." The California Legislative Counsel defines a spot bill as a bill that amends a code section in such an innocuous way as to be totally nonsubstantive. The bill has been introduced to assure that a germane vehicle will be available at a later date after the deadline has passed to introduce bills. It appears that SB 289, sponsored by the California Hospital Association, may propose an expansion of eligibility to the classes of hospitals granted 2 year extensions by SB 1661.

6.4 A Decade of Angst and Adjustments

The decade from 2000 to 2010 was marked by a large number of efforts to make adjustments to a program experiencing seriously lagging implementation resulting from an almost endless array of complications. For the entire decade, more than half California's hospitals were experiencing extraordinary financial constraints. Despite the fact that OSPHD's SB 1953 review staff was paid entirely by fees from hospitals, the agency was prohibited from hiring additional staff because of a state hiring freeze and, to make matters worse, was also required to participate in the State's employee furlough program – a program in which state employees were required to take a specified number of days off at no pay. This, coupled with greater design complexity than was originally envisaged, resulted in hospital plan reviews taking much longer than anyone had anticipated. Construction costs continued to increase as the cost of materials escalated much more rapidly than general inflation. It was a long, difficult decade that resulted in significantly slower compliance with SB 1953 than either the seismic safety advocates or OSHPD had anticipated.

In 2001, two of the authors had lunch with an OSHPD staff member who will remain anonymous. After reviewing the magnitude of the challenges SB 1953 posed for OSHPD, this official said something to us that characterized the early years of implementation for program and hospital administrators alike: "All roads lead to 'we're screwed'."

Throughout the decade, while willing to provide extensions to hospitals to achieve compliance, the legislature was steadfastly unwilling to provide financial assistance or non-cash incentives to hospitals to upgrade or replace their facilities.

6.4.1 An Updated Compliance Calendar

Four extensions to the initial compliance deadlines for SB 1953 were enacted between the time the Act was passed and 2010 (Fig. 6.1). The first of these, SB 1801 provided a very limited number of hospitals with year by year extensions of the 2008 provisions for up to 5 years. SB 1801 permitted specified, contiguous hospital buildings an extension of the 2008 deadline if the hospital agreed that the designated services would be provided by moving into an existing conforming building, relocating to a new building, or retrofitting the existing building to meet the 2030 standards. OSHPD reports that only two facilities obtained extensions under SB 1801 to the year 2013 (Carlisle and Coleman 2010).

The second extension was SB 1661. It extended the time for bringing SPC-1 buildings into compliance to 2015 for hospitals that were actively working on compliance but whose projects were delayed because of circumstances beyond their control.

Third, SB 306 enabled hospitals with serious financial problems to receive extensions from complying with upgrading, replacing, or removing acute care services from SPC-1 buildings if they agreed to replace the structures by 2020 rather than 2030. OSHPD reported that, as of 2010, only 24 hospitals received extensions (Carlisle and Coleman 2010, p. 16).

The final extension was embodied in SB 499 which permitted OSHPD to use HAZUS to reassess SPC-1 buildings for seismic resistance and to raise the collapse threshold from 0.75% probability of collapse to 1.2% probability of collapse. SB 499 also expanded eligibility for SB 1661 extensions.

6.5 Where Things Stood at the End of 2010 and into 2011

6.5.1 Compliance

In March, 2010, OSHPD's Director, David M. Carlisle, and Deputy Director for Facilities Development, Paul A. Coleman, presented testimony to the California Senate Health Committee at its Hearing on Hospital Seismic Safety in which they provided a history of SB 1953, changes to the legislation, and an extensive and detailed account of hospital compliance with SB 1953 (Carlisle and Coleman 2010).

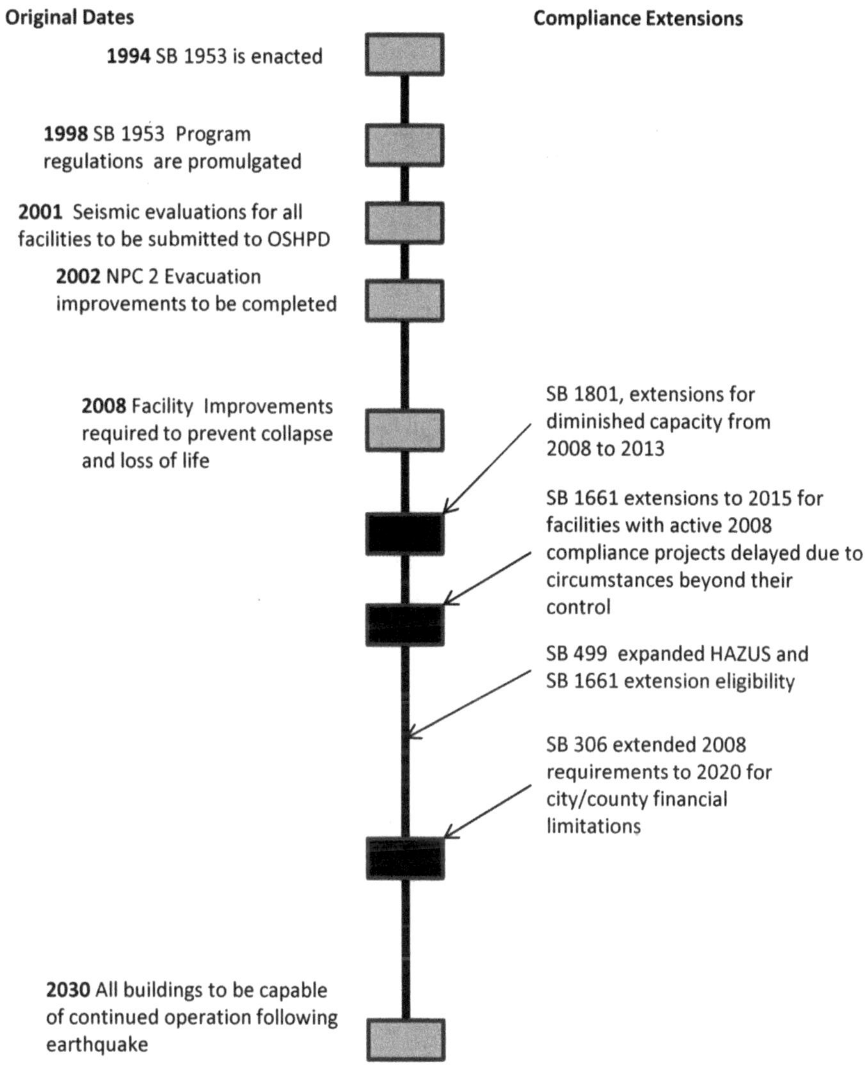

Fig. 6.1 Original and revised compliance dates for SPC-1 hospital buildings under SB 1953, as amended (Source: California Senate Health Committee Hearing on Hospital Seismic Safety, March 3, 2010. Testimony by the Office of Statewide Health Planning and Development (OSHPD))

They reported that of the 1,027 hospital buildings that were classified as SPC-1 in 2001, 825 remained as SPC-1 buildings as of January, 2010. That means that, between 2001 and 2010, 202 of the 1027 buildings classified as subject to collapse in a major earthquake were brought into compliance. Compliance was achieved by retrofitting the noncompliant building, by taking it out of use as an acute care facility, or through reevaluation moving the building to an SPC-2 classification. Unfortunately, that number amounts to slightly less than 20% of the buildings originally classified in

Table 6.2 OSHPD summary of SB 1953 compliance as of January 2010, including estimated effects of SB 499, March 2010

Total hospital buildings in 2001	2627
Total SPC-1 hospital buildings in 2001	1027
Hospital buildings brought into compliance 2001–2009	202
Total remaining SPC-1 hospital buildings in 2009	825
Hospital buildings likely to comply with SB 1661	632
Estimated SPC-1 buildings remaining	≈ 193
Hospital buildings likely to be reclassified by HAZUS as SPC-2 in 2010	≈ 48
Estimated SPC-1 hospital buildings remaining	≈ 145

Source: California Senate Health Committee Hearing on Hospital Seismic Safety, Testimony by the Office of Statewide Health Planning and Development, March 2, 2010, page 28

2001 as being in danger of collapse from an earthquake and scheduled for achieving compliance by January, 2008.

On the other hand, 326 of the 825 remaining buildings "presently have active compliance projects and are expected to be retrofitted or replaced by 2013" (Carlisle and Coleman 2010, p. 19). Of the 825, 74 have SB 306 extensions to 2020. Another 142 buildings are expected to be withdrawn from service by 2013 and 39 buildings have active projects that will be replaced by 2015 if they receive SB 1661 extensions.

Table 6.2, *OSHPD Summary of SB 1953 Compliance as of January 2010, Including Estimated Effects of SB 499, March 2010,* details where the agency saw SPC-1 hospitals in terms of compliance with SB 1953 as amended by the extensions granted in legislation since 1998. The information in the table paints a relatively bright picture of the number of hospitals complying with the law. Of the 825 SPC-1 buildings remaining as acute care facilities in 2009, 632 are expected to comply with SB 1661, meaning the hospitals have until 2015 to being them into compliance. Of the 193 remaining SPC-1 buildings, about 48 are expected to be reclassified in 2010 as SPC-2 buildings and not require replacement until 2030. Only 145 buildings remain as SPC-1 hospitals not in compliance with SB 1953.

By 2010, people in those buildings originally classified in 2002 as SPC-1 were, for the most part, somewhat safer than they had been before SB 1953 was enacted. No one in any of those buildings that were converted from acute care to other hospital uses without any retrofitting was any safer. Virtually all of those buildings that remained in acute care use completed the requirements due in 2002 for nonstructural improvements. Failure of nonstructural components was a primary reason for hospitals being unable to operate continuously following earthquakes. It was essential to upgrade those buildings to help ensure safety from falling equipment and to facilitate building evacuation. Nonetheless, relatively few hospital facilities had actually been upgraded or replaced to meet the structural standards that were supposed to have been put in place as of January 2008. As of January 2008, hospitals owned by cities, counties, special districts, and the University of California had the highest proportion of their buildings (72%) still classified as SPC-1, contrasted with 53% of investor-owned hospital buildings. Some buildings achieved compliance by obtaining extensions for extenuating circumstances and others were able to be reclassified as SPC-2 by virtue of reanalysis under the HAZUS provisions.

By February, 2011, OSHPD had become optimistic about the extent of hospital compliance with SB 1953.

> The preliminary results of a recently completed statewide survey indicated that more than 80 percent of California hospitals with buildings considered at risk during a major earthquake will meet new safety standards by 2015. This is good new for patients, hospital employees, and local communities alike (Dauner 2011).

There is, of course, a significant difference between being in compliance with the provisions of SB 1953 and having met the substantive requirements of structural and nonstructural seismic safety specified in the Act. Hundreds of hospital buildings were "defined" into compliance because their special circumstances or because the more sophisticated screening system (HAZUS) led to their reclassification as SPC-2 buildings that would not have to be replaced until 2030. When all is said and done, few buildings classified as SPC-1 in 2001 met the January 1, 2008 deadline for compliance with SB 1953. By November 2008, 116 buildings had been reclassified as SPC-2 buildings (Degenkolb 2010) and additional reclassifications since then have significantly increased the number of reclassified buildings.

Even though OSHPD's statement that about 80% of the hospitals classified as most dangerous will be being in compliance by 2015 is technically accurate, it seems to us to be misleading to suggest or imply that people in those hospitals are safer because SB 1953 resulted in widespread retrofit and replacement. Obviously, some of them will have been retrofitted and replaced by 2015. With that construction, the State's deadline extensions for others, and the reclassifications made employing HAZUS, the State has been able to put a good face on a difficult situation.

6.5.2 *Unanticipated Consequences*

Few public policies are implemented without unanticipated, often adverse, side effects. SB 1953 has had its share of adverse side effects. Primary among these are: contributing to the financial problems of a healthcare industry in turmoil, the financial insolvency of a few hospitals, reduced access to healthcare in low income areas, and contributing to moving staff and nonacute care patients into buildings classified by the State as subject to collapse in an earthquake.

6.5.2.1 Closures and Reduced Service Availability in Lower Income Areas

Many California hospitals closed between 1998 and 2010. The Nicholas C. Petris Center found that 23 acute care hospitals closed from 1995 through 2001 (Nicholas C. Petris Center 2001). Closures continued after 2001. The California Healthcare Foundation reported that, since 2001, "27 hospitals closed, resulting in a loss of about 3,500 beds. Forty-one percent of these hospitals and 58% of the beds were in

Los Angeles County. During the same period, six hospitals opened with 373 beds" (California Health Care 2010). Closures in the Los Angeles area accounted for 41% of all closures and 58% of beds removed from service between 2001 and 2007. The new hospitals added were not in the same locations as those that closed.

The most significant number of hospital closures occurred coincident with the enactment and implementation of SB 1953. Does this mean that SB 1953 was a major factor in those closures? Correlation, of course, does not imply causality. The reasons for closures were complex and varied; it appears that almost all of the closures were associated with rising costs, declining reimbursements, and an increase in bad debts and charity cases. These closures were driven by financial problems including the looming need for retrofit and ultimate replacement. Unfortunately, most of the closures were in areas where they were needed desperately. SB 1953 probably contributed to the closure of some general acute care hospitals in California; the pending costs of retrofit or of rebuilding may well have been the straw that broke the camel's back.

It is unlikely that SB 1953 led to the closure of any hospital that was financially sound with good prospects for continued viability at the time SB 1953 was enacted.

The closure of so many privately-owned hospitals in low income areas placed a greatly increased burden for caring for the uninsured and indigent on hospitals owned by local and state government and obliged to remain in operation to provide service.

A very important series of closings was not associated with SB 1953. This was the closing of a large number of emergency centers in acute care hospitals. Hospitals with emergency rooms are required by law to serve everyone who comes to their facility requiring emergency care, regardless of their ability to pay. As each emergency care center closed, the burden on nearby hospitals with emergency rooms increased, creating additional financial problems for them.

6.5.2.2 Others Were Placed in Danger

One of the responses by hospital owners to comply with the SB 1953 was to remove acute care use from noncompliant structures, Often, though, the hospital owners to put that building to some other use. This presumably made those who moved out from the noncompliant buildings safer, but, at the same time, it put those who were moved into those buildings either no safer or in greater danger. We have been unable to determine how many acute care hospital buildings classified as SPC-1 were converted from acute care to some other use without significantly altering the building's seismic resistance. We know the number is significant. The buildings are now used to house administrative or medical staff, student nurses, patients with chronic illness, or other hospital uses not defined as acute care.

An important question arises from this practice and from the law that triggered the behavior. Why are patients and staff who occupy acute care facilities more deserving of being in a building that is seismically safer than are out-patients, nursing students, mental health patients, administrators, and other hospital staff and patients? The answer appears to be simply in the way the framers of the policy perceived and defined the problem. They believed that "Hospitals must remain standing and functional during and after an earthquake for the safety of patients and staff AND (emphasis in original) to provide medical assistance to earthquake victims" (OSHPD 2005).

Since no provision was made for enhancing the seismic safety of patients and staff outside of acute care facilities, one must conclude that the policy's framers were concerned primarily with the ability of the hospital facility to continue operations following an earthquake to help victims and less concerned with the safety of existing patients and non-emergency medical staff. That, in turn, raises the question as to whether there might be significantly more cost-effective approaches to achieve the objective of ensuring prompt and appropriate medical care to earthquake victims, such as the use of temporary emergency triage areas outside the hospital buildings.

6.6 In Retrospect: A Well-Intended Intervention with Unfortunate Unanticipated Outcomes

In the immediate aftermath of the 1906 San Francisco earthquake, community boosters who saw pride, progress, and profit stemming from community growth promoted the idea that the earthquake was simply an anomaly and that the real culprit in the city's demolition was the fire that followed it. By the time of the 1933 Long Beach earthquake, Californians had started to understand they lived in earthquake country and they began to take steps to protect themselves by enacting increasingly rigorous building codes. The Great Depression and World War II essentially put a hold on most efforts to enhance seismic safety, but as damaging earthquakes were experienced in the 1970s and more recently, the State government took steps to retrofit or rebuild elements of the infrastructure that had proven to be vulnerable to seismic forces. Freeway bridges and overpasses were retrofitted to enhance seismic resistance. New utility life lines (gas, electricity, etc.) were designed to be more robust and existing lifelines were strengthened. As California State Government worked its way through the list of important community assets in need of strengthening, hospitals became a matter of some concern. As we have already seen, the legislature, under the leadership of Senator Alquist, enacted increasingly stringent codes for new hospital construction beginning in 1973. As we have also seen, seismic safety advocates became increasingly concerned about the safety of hospitals built before 1973 and the slow rate at which they appeared to be replaced by new, safer structures.

From this standpoint, SB 1953 can be seen as simply the next logical item in a long agenda of steps intended to make California's critical facilities safer from earthquakes. As it turns out, however, achieving the retrofit or replacement of older hospitals proved to be much more of a challenge than seismic safety advocates had imagined.

Who could possibly disagree with the need to have acute care hospitals sufficiently resistant to earthquakes so that patients and staff would be safe and so that they could continue to function following the earthquake, treating existing patients and those injured in the earthquake? It is difficult to imagine that anyone other than someone with serious mental or emotional problems could be opposed. As with most things, the devil was in the details. While most could agree with the goal, disagreements arose over who should bear the costs, relative priorities, and what some saw as intractable obstacles to goal attainment.

SB 1953 was intended to ensure that all acute care hospitals in California would meet high standards for seismic safety by 2030. Hospitals with nonstructural deficiencies would meet a set of intermediate goals quickly and hospital facilities with structural deficiencies would meet various levels of seismic resistance based on a timetable which, to those who supported the legislation, seemed entirely reasonable. It didn't work out quite as expected, especially in the early years. The most dangerous facilities were to have been retrofitted, replaced, or taken from acute care use by 2008. That date came and went without much in the way of substantive compliance. Deferrals were given to many individual facilities for a variety of reasons. Some observers predict that 2030 will come and go without full compliance. The program has placed extraordinary costs and burdens on most hospitals that require attention; in 2007, the costs of compliance were put at about $169 billion. Adverse unanticipated consequences include the program contributing to the closure of many hospitals, particularly in low income, underserved areas. As a consequence, a program that was intended to help ensure the availability of treatment *after* an earthquake has contributed to some unknown extent to reducing the availability of treatment *both before and after* an earthquake.

Thus far, the outcomes are mixed. A senior structural engineer who had supported the legislation and with whom we spoke many times lamented that "We thought we were doing a good thing – the right thing." A few cynics we talked with disagree, but we believe that those who supported the legislation and worked for its enactment were well-intentioned and sincere in their belief that the program would address a serious, urgent problem. Alas, that is too often the case. Well-meaning, knowledgeable people promote solutions to persistent problems and those solutions, when enacted, often have undesirable side effects. In our business, it is often called the Law of Unanticipated Consequences, a term framed and popularized early in the twentieth century, it is said, by sociologist Robert K. Merton. Unanticipated consequences can be favorable, unfavorable, or actually exacerbate the problem the policy was intended to mitigate.

Certainly, SB 1953 has contributed significantly to a new hospital building boom in California. Few hospital owners have chosen to retrofit buildings constructed before 1973 and that makes good sense. Most of those facilities are not very compatible with modern medical practice and the need for greater efficiency. Moderate earthquakes are fairly common in California and a strong earthquake is quite likely to occur within many hospital buildings' normal lifespan. Thus, it is likely that actions taken in response to SB 1953 will prevent some deaths and injuries between now and 2030. Those who championed the law will then be able to point with pride to benefits of the Act. Nonetheless, the cost of taking the old hospitals out from the inventory and putting new facilities in their place has proven to be extraordinary, even excluding the opportunity costs. The fact that hospitals were in desperate financial circumstances at the exact time they were mandated to enhance their seismic safety was quite unfortunate. We will leave it to others to draw conclusions about whether the benefits will warrant the costs.

6.7 Looking Ahead

In 2009, a senior executive with a major California-based structural engineering firm active in helping hospitals comply with SB 1953 observed that,

> The economy and credit crisis today are pressuring hospitals to delay, downsize, or cancel construction projects and major equipment purchases. With capital markets tightening, more than 25 percent of hospitals are unable to acquire financing for construction projects. The California Hospital Association reports that an estimated 41 percent of hospitals halted construction projects or major equipment purchases and 40 percent forecast that they will not be able to meet the seismic upgrade requirements by the 2013 and 2015 intermediate deadlines. The growing number of uninsured patients, record losses in unpaid medical bills, and the loss of investment holdings have further crippled hospitals' abilities to meet the mandate (Poland 2010).

OSHPD, too, recognized the continuing financial problems facing many California hospitals. OSHPD reports that,

> 70 % of hospitals report deterioration in the investment holdings, 25 % of hospital (sic) are unable to secure capital for seismic upgrades, 41% of hospitals have halted work on construction projects, 38 % of hospitals have reported they cannot make 2013 or 2015 upgrade deadlines, (and) hospitals absorb $10 billion in providing care to charity and indigent (Borba 2009).

SB 1953 was only one among many contributing factors creating widespread financial problems for California hospitals. There is little doubt, however, that as a significant number of hospitals with extensions to 2013, 2015, 2020, and 2030 approach those deadlines, the financial impact of SB 1953 may become far more salient and far larger. A case from December 2001 may be illustrative.

The Henry Mayo Memorial Hospital in Valencia was damaged in the 1994 Northridge Earthquake. The not-for-profit hospital spent $35 million to repair the facility and to retrofit it to meet the then-existing 2008 deadline for structural compliance. The hospital received $23 million from FEMA and from insurance claims, leaving a $12 million gap. The hospital drew the $12 million from its capital pool, but was left with very little flexibility to meet subsequent contingencies. A major contingent event occurred shortly after the repairs were completed. A series of agreements with health insurers did not work out at all well and the hospital ended up filing for Chap. 11 bankruptcy protection (Darmiento 2001). The story is apparently ending well. A review of Cal-Mortgage financial reports indicates that the hospital, the only general acute care hospital in rapidly growing Santa Clarita

County in 2001, is still in operation. As of June 30, 2009, it had outstanding loan guarantees of about $125 million but is classified by Cal-Mortgage as "having no problems" with servicing the debt (OSHPD 2009)

In the first 12 years following the promulgation of the SB 1953 program regulations, few hospitals were retrofitted or replaced. Compliance has been achieved primarily by reclassifying buildings as safer than originally classified and by providing extensions for entirely legitimate purposes. We expect that compliance will continue to lag and that extensions to deadlines will continue to be enacted, perhaps even beyond 2030, only 20 years from now. We expect this because at least half of California's hospitals with old buildings continue to experience serious financial problems and building new hospitals continues to become increasingly more expensive. It will be necessary to wait to see how the hospitals with continuing financial problems address SB 1953 compliance as the deadlines for structural compliance for each of them approaches.

We do not expect the California State government to provide financial support to hospitals attempting to upgrade their facilities, nor do we expect hospitals with financial resources to acquire hospitals in impoverished communities unless financial incentives are enacted and the requirements to treat the uninsured and indigent without cost are changed. Compliance will become more problematic as the hospitals that can find ways to rebuild remove themselves from the noncompliance pool and those remaining in the noncompliance pool increasingly constitute the most impoverished hospitals.

We are not encouraged by some of the outcomes we have seen over the past decade or so. It appears that the "haves" are gaining access to new hospital buildings with enhanced seismic safety and more contemporary treatment facilities, while the "have nots" find themselves increasingly forced to travel greater distances for emergency, out-patient, and in-patient care in overcrowded facilities that are unlikely to be able to maintain operations following a significant earthquake. In this sense, implementing SB 1953 cannot be viewed separately from the increasingly intractable problems associated with healthcare for the poor and uninsured, increasing costs of healthcare, and what we see as increasingly difficult competitive challenges for hospitals in the face of diminishing compensation from Medicare, government medical assistance to the poor, and insurers.

We do, nonetheless, expect that SB 1953 will result in all of California's acute care hospital facilities being brought into compliance with the standards embodied in that policy. We are not convinced that it will happen by 2030; it is likely that more changes will be made to the compliance schedule as conditions continue to change and as new concerns arise. Our expectations are tempered by the high probability that a significant earthquake will occur between now and 2030, damaging hospitals, perhaps resulting in deaths in an old hospital facility, the inability to treat some of the injured, and a subsequent impetus from the public and government to get the replacements done quickly. Unless that were to happen, we expect a continuation of the kinds of extensions that have been granted to hospitals facing various circumstances. The most recent of these occurred in April 2011, when the legislature adopted SB 90 as amended. Among other things, the new law grants individual hospitals the ability to apply for an extension of deadlines for seismic compliance of up to 7 years, and authorizes the Office of State Health Planning and Development to grant an extension provided the hospital meets certain conditions. The law will result in extending the compliance deadline for some of the hospitals that were to be retrofit, replaced, or taken from service in 2013–2020. The law was sponsored by the California Hospital Association and is opposed by the California Nurses Association. The law is roughly comparable to other modifications to compliance deadlines made, essentially, since SB 1953 regulations were promulgated. We fully expect more of the same until 2030 and perhaps beyond.

References

Barnard M (2010) Cited in what hospitals can do. Perspectives. Degenkolb, San Francisco, May 2010

Borba DF (2009) OSHPD regulatory update, hospital building safety board, quarterly meeting, 9–10 Nov 2009, Duane F. Borba, P.E., Acting Deputy Division Chief, Facilities Development Division

California Health Care Foundation (2010) California hospitals facts and figures. Health Care Almanac, Sacramento, April 2010

California State Senate (2006) Senate bill no. 1661, an act to amend Section 130060 of, and to add Section 130061 to, the health and safety code, relating to health facilities. California State Senate, Sacramento

California State Senate (2009) Senate bill no. 499, an act to amend Section 130060 and 130061 of, and to repeal Section 130022 of the health and safety code, relating to health facilities. California State Senate, Sacramento

California State Senate Health Committee (2007) SB 306 bill analysis. California State Senate Health Committee, Sacramento

California State Senate Health Committee (2009) SB 499 bill analysis. California State Senate Health Committee, Sacramento

Cal-Mortgage (2010) Loan insurance legislative reports, report 1 – financial status of borrowers, 2009 financial status report. Office of Statewide Health Planning and Development, Sacramento

Carlisle DM, Coleman PA (2010) California Senate Health Committee hearing on hospital seismic safety, 17 Feb 2010. Testimony by The Office of Statewide Health Planning and Development

Darmiento L (2001) Hospital's Woes Demonstrate Perils of Retrofit Mandate. Los Angel Bus J, http://www.labusinessjournal.com, 10 Dec 2001

Dauner CD (2011) California hospitals making good progress. California Hospital Association. http://www.calhospital.or/oshpd-survey, 1 Feb 2011

Gillengarten J, Tokas C (2008) Reassessment and reprioritization program for SPC-1 hospital buildings: overview of the reassessment program – why HAZUS? PowerPoint presentation prepared by the Office of Statewide Health Planning and Development

Greene J (2006) Climbing construction cost. Hospital and Health Networks Digital Magazine (H &HN). Published exclusively online (www.hhnmag.com) vol. 19, p. 5

Marois MB (2008) California bond yields rise to four-year high on budget impasse. http://www.bloomberg.com 26 Dec 2008

Meade C, Kulick J (2007) SB 1953 and the challenge of hospital seismic safety in California. Prepared for the California HealthCare Foundation (Sacramento, CA) by RAND (Santa Monica, CA) January 2007

Nicholas C. Petris Center (2001) California's closed hospitals, 1995–2000. Nicholas C. Petris Center on Health Care markets and consumer welfare, April. University of California, Berkeley, School of Public Health, Berkeley

OSHPD (2005) California's hospital seismic safety law: its history, implementation, & progress. Office of Statewide Healthcare Planning and Development, Sacramento

OSHPD (2009). Annual report to the California legislature on the financial status of the California health facility construction loan insurance program and insured portfolio for the fiscal year ending 30 June 2009. Office of Statewide Healthcare Planning and Development, Sacramento

Poland C (2010) Cited in *The Issue at Hand.* Perspectives. Degenkolb, San Francisco, May 2010

Part II
Obstacles to Implementation: The Usual Suspects

Most of the literature focuses on impediments to public policy implementation in terms of the roles and behaviors of agencies that implement those policies and on related matters such as the intricacies of intergovernmental sharing of responsibilities. This specific case involves only one agency, that being OSHPD, the state agency charged with administering the provisions of SB 1953. To be sure, a host of other state agencies were involved in one way to another and each, to some extent, had an impact on implementation. Nevertheless, analysis of the state's program administrators does not appear to corroborate any conclusions that agency behaviors are the principal impediment to the long and difficult road to SB 1953 implementation. It is necessary to look beyond the usual suspects.

Chapter 7
OSHPD, Administrative Agencies in General, and Implementing SB 1953

7.1 Introduction

As stated previously, our focus is on adding to our collective understanding of public policy implementation as it relates to reducing the likely consequences of extreme events, including, particularly, natural hazard events. The SB 1953 experience provides an excellent example of a policy that has been achieving its stated objectives slowly and gradually, but, unfortunately, not without adverse and largely unanticipated consequences.

We have concluded that there are many reasons why things have unfolded as they have. Historically, when public policies and programs have not worked out quite as anticipated, analysts have looked within government to learn what went wrong. Most of the implementation literature examines what happens within and between government agencies in terms of how they administer programs intended to foster one or another outcome. The focus is the agencies charged with administering the policies and with the nexus and tangencies of the various agencies charged with one or another aspect of implementation.

Regulatory policy, though, is a form of public policy that calls for government organizations to do things to induce *others* to take the actions intended to achieve the ends toward which the policy is directed. Regulatory policy, by its very nature, comprises two critical sets of actors: those whose job it is to induce others to take action to comply with the requirement, and those organizations whose actions are the target of the policy.

This chapter focuses on the first half of the equation: factors affecting the performance of the agency or agencies charged with administering the policy intended to induce other organizations to take action. Later chapters will address the actions taken by the organizations targeted by the policy.

D.J. Alesch et al., *Natural Hazard Mitigation Policy: Implementation, Organizational Choice, and Contextual Dynamics*, Environmental Hazards, DOI 10.1007/978-94-007-2235-4_7, © Springer Science+Business Media B.V. 2012

7.2 OSHPD: Mission, Culture, and Perspectives

The mission of OSHPD clearly communicates its purpose and primary activities:

> The Mission of (the) Office of Statewide Health Planning and Development (OSHPD) is to promote healthcare accessibility through leadership in analyzing California's healthcare infrastructure, promoting a diverse and competent healthcare workforce, providing information about healthcare outcomes, assuring the safety of buildings used in providing healthcare, insuring loans to encourage the development of healthcare facilities, and facilitating development of sustained capacity for communities to address local healthcare issues (OSHPD 2011).

Perhaps more so than its mission, OSHPD's stated values lend insight into its approach to SB 1953. Its values, abbreviated here, include:

1. Accountability. As a government agency, we are held accountable for our actions. In fact, this accountability is one of the prime factors that separates governmental from private sector organizations. … This accountability generates certain expectations for our actions.
2. Service. OSHPD is essentially a service organization, providing services for our clients. … We are recognized for the quality and consistency of the services that we provide. Maintaining and even improving upon this level of achievement is a demanding but achievable goal.
3. Communication. Communication means that it is important for the Office to effectively and reliably transmit information both internally and externally.
4. Innovation typifies what we do at OSHPD.
5. Integrity. This is a very important value for a governmental organization. The dictionary includes the definition: firm adherence to a code of especially moral or artistic values, i.e. incorruptibility. At OSHPD, with regard to both our internal operations and external relationships, Integrity also means that we can be counted on to always perform in a consistent and fair manner.
6. Professionalism means high standards, self-accountability, and responsibility. Other identified characteristics of professionalism include the need to maintain an on-going educational process, dedication, and awareness of professional norms in order to achieve a consistency of performance. Put another way, OSHPD professionals can be relied upon to always perform in a uniformly excellent manner by continually improving their capabilities and competencies.
7. Respect. Respect is a value that OSHPD staff use to guide their work on a daily basis. Respect has meaning for both internal and external relationships with our constituents. … OSHPD has rarely (indeed almost never) received complaints about the way the office treats its clients.
8. Teamwork. OSHPD works as a team of many teams. A team-based approach allows us to synergistically apply our various strengths and technical competencies.

An organization's culture is "the pattern of shared basic assumptions learned by a group as it solves its problems of external adaptation and internal integration" (Schein 2010, p. 18). Organizational culture has both visible and assumed elements.

Visible elements include statements of espoused values, such as those described on the OSHPD website. These values are intended to guide decision making by organizational members and also to inform relevant stakeholders, such as the general public, about what matters to a given organization.

In the case of OSHPD, one might describe its culture as being role oriented (Harrison 1979) or bureaucratic. Such cultures emphasize consistency, efficiency, and stability over innovation and responsiveness. This isn't intended to imply that OSHPD is not responsive. Rather, the focus of OSHPD is consistency in operations rather than say, inventiveness. Innovation is not ignored, but accountability is first priority, and accountability demands consistency in operations. Interaction is formalized, with standard operating procedures dictating processes. Strategic decisions and their means of implementation flow from the top of the organization to the bottom. Tasks are specialized. Departments engage with one another through formal means.

Role cultures and their accompanying structural elements enable consistency over variability. In the case of an agency such as OSHPD, one should not be surprised by its emphasis on *accountability* as a first value. After all, it is a government agency beholden to taxpayers and their myriad and sometimes conflicting expectations. A common expectation is that *services* will be consistently delivered, and that no one will be treated inequitably. Ensuring fair treatment across a wide range and high number of users typically leads to the creation of standardized procedures and forms. Trying to anticipate how the wide range and high number of users might read and comprehend the standard operating procedures and forms often leads to lengthy forms (and forms to understand the forms) that are vetted by legal staff to minimize the potential for misunderstanding and litigation. Producing and approving such forms, and training staff on their use, can take considerable time. Once the forms are labeled and in regular use, it becomes difficult to behave in nonstandard ways. And hence the bureaucracy, or red tape, that many people jest and complain about, is created and nurtured.

OSHPD lists *integrity* as one of its values. As with accountability and service, integrity as a value supports the role oriented or bureaucratic culture that enables OSHPD to perform its functions. Likewise, *professionalism* encourages OSHPD staff members to "always perform in a uniformly excellent manner." It's clear that OSHPD takes its responsibilities seriously and wants to serve the taxpaying public to the very best of its staff members' abilities. It is able to cite many examples of its ability and willingness to meet stakeholders' expectations.

One of the potentially negative aspects of a role oriented culture is that the push for consistently excellent service can lead to an overabundance of standard operating procedures and an unwillingness to review and occasionally dispense with historically useful procedures. A desire to behave in consistent ways can make innovation difficult. Importantly, OSHPD also lists innovation as one of its values, suggesting that it understands and tries to address the tension between consistency and responsiveness. This is likely an area that challenges OSHPD's staff members, as the pressure to continually and consistently perform in certain ways tends to constrain proposed (and unproven) changes intended to enhance operations and service.

7.3 The Usual Suspects: Main Threads in the Literature About Administrative Agencies and Implementation

Because so much of the implementation literature focuses on the agencies charged with program administration, it is incumbent on us to examine the role of OSHPD, the agency charged with implementing SB 1953. We assessed the SB 1953 experience to ascertain the extent to which OSHPD helped or hindered policy implementation. We did so, in part, by looking what the literature has to say about implementation and the "usual suspects" – government's administrative agencies – and how it relates to OSHPD and the SB 1953 experience. Given what we learned in the case study, we also look to see what the literature fails to say.

The policy implementation literature is rich with research findings on relationships between the internal workings of governments on implementation effectiveness. From this literature, we selected several variables we thought most closely fit the circumstances of this case as it relates to program administration.

7.3.1 Complexity: The Number of Participating Agencies and Levels of Government and Checkpoints in the Process

The organizational environment within which a public organization attempts to implement a program is critically important to successful implementation. As far back as 1973, Pressman and Wildavsky (1973) concluded that a multiplicity of participants and perspectives combine to produce formidable obstacles to implementation. They concluded that when a program depends on many actors, there are numerous possibilities for disagreement and delay and that, given a large number of clearance points manned by diverse and independent participants, the probability of a program achieving its goals is low. We agree. The probability of successful, timely implementation of natural hazard mitigation policies is inversely related with the complexity of the policy and implementation process, the number of actors participating in the process, the number of sign-offs required, and the diversity of interests and priorities among the actors.

We were able to eliminate from our analysis the literature that addresses problems of policy drift that often occurs when agencies at various levels of government are involved in implementing a single policy. The complexity of that phenomenon is avoided in this analysis because only one level of government was involved – the State of California – and only one agency – OSHPD – had responsibility for program administration. This allowed us to focus on other implementation obstacles without having to consider how we might control for a complex implementation network.

7.3.2 Congruence Between Agency Culture and the Policy

The literature leads us to believe that policies are more likely to be implemented successfully when they are entrusted for implementation to organizations that embrace the same goals and values as those implicit or explicit in the policy. Alesch and Petak (2001), for example, concluded that the probability of successful implementation increases to the extent that actors in the implementation process perceive congruence between means and ends; that is, they will work harder to ensure implementation if they perceive that the policy and the programs designed to implement the policy are appropriate, given their perception of the problem.

One would expect greater commitment to implementing a policy if it is congruent with organizational culture and with the values, beliefs, and focus of organizational leaders and staff. When a policy is enacted that is not congruent with the value set or expectations or desires of those expected to implement it, then it is essentially sending a directive into the dense medium of the bureaucracy where it is likely to wither. Sabatier and Mazmanian (1979) argue that implementation will proceed more directly when implementation is assigned to agencies that are supportive of statutory objectives. They will give the new program high priority. Similarly, successful implementation is more likely with the decision rules of the implementing agencies are supportive of policy objectives.

The SB 1953 legislation was fully congruent with the OSHPD mission and, based on our discussions over the years with OSHPD staff, it was entirely congruent with agency culture and the perspective of agency administrators. Agency staffers, in collaboration with the Hospital Building Safety Board (HBSB), wrote the program regulations that operationalized SB 1953 and OSHPD promulgated the rules after they had been approved by the California Building Standards Board, a separate agency.

Based on our analysis, we do not believe there was a lack of congruence between OSHPD's culture and values and the policy that might contribute to obstacles to program implementation. We certainly did not observe any and none were reported to us by knowledgeable observers.

7.3.3 Organizational Capacity and Capability

Sometimes organizations that are committed fully to a policy or program find themselves short of the resources needed to expeditiously proceed with program implementation. We concur with Sabatier and Mazmanian (1979) that implementation is more likely to be successful if sufficient resources are made available to the implementing agencies for hiring staff, developing regulations, administering and permit and service delivery programs, and monitoring compliance by the target group. May and Williams (1986), examining federal agency involvement in natural hazard mitigation programs, observe that federal agencies themselves have problems focusing on mitigation programs because of capacity issues. Godschalk and colleagues (1999) agree, stating that capacity as well as program commitment are key variables.

Organizational capacity refers to the resources available to the organization to apply toward program implementation. Resources include all those elements necessary to achieve implementation, including both resource quality and quantity. Among the essential resources are an adequate number of persons with sufficient talent to carry out the activities necessary for implementation. Resources include, too, sufficient time to implement the program, sufficient financial support, sufficient technology, and sufficient authority to do what is required. Organizational capacity also includes attention span. Organizations with an overloaded agenda, working under pressure, are unlikely to be able to give enough attention to a new program to mount a successful effort unless that program has an exceptionally high priority. Even then, without sufficient resources, agencies fully committed to implementation have difficulty performing up to expectations.

OSHPD experienced extremely heavy workloads as hospital owners and their architectural and engineering consultants began to request additional information, clarifications, and plan reviews. The organization was insufficiently staffed to keep pace with the demands by program generated. The agency requested authorization to hire additional staff, but the State of California was suffering financial problems and had frozen new hires. Even though the additional OSHPD employees would have been funded entirely by fees paid by those submitting plans, the requests for additional staffing were denied. The State's refusal to make an exception to the hiring freeze in OSHPD's case had an adverse effect on the ability of OSHPD to keep pace with the demands being placed upon it by regulated parties seeking to comply with the law. In turn, the regulated parties were delayed in complying with the law.

The agency was eventually able to gain some flexibility in adapting to the inevitable glitches that accompany initiating a new program; it became clear that the program needed to be modified to deal with problems that emerged during the early stages of implementation. OSHPD requested and received approval that its programmatic changes would be processed by the external approval body as emergency changes rather than as routine changes. This resulted in a significant reduction in the time required to get approval of changes and facilitated the agency's ability to administer the program.

7.3.4 "Street Level" Staffing, Complexity, and Judgment

For decades, implementation analysts have considered the characteristics and behavior of the staff that has direct contact with parties targeted by public policies and programs as it affects successful program administration (Lipsky 1971; May and Wood 2003). Lipsky (1971) referred to those having direct contact with parties targeted by a program as street level bureaucrats. Most of the political science literature that addresses obstacles to effective implementation looks at multi-level, multi-organizational systems and does not apply in this case.

We gave relatively little attention to the matter of interactions between "street level" implementors and "clients" and were unable to assess the extent to which such interactions had any effect on implementation. We heard considerable grousing from both OSHPD staff and from engineers seeking plan reviews and approvals about each other. Each of the authors has been in both the position of the one doing the reviewing and the position of the one wanting the review quickly and accurately; hence, we judged that the squabbles were of a fairly normal quality and quantity.

Our talks with participants suggested that most of the interchanges were entirely civil, but that, as is so often the case in regulatory processes, after the meetings, one or another or both parties were dissatisfied with the outcome.

The literature is not silent on the matter of complexity, but it focuses more on complexity of institutional arrangements and the number of participants in a process than it does on the inherent programmatic complexity. The SB 1953 program and regulations address complex phenomena relating to structural design and performance. Not every contingency can (or should be) covered by program regulations, so there is, by necessity, some ambiguity about how this or that regulation might apply to one or another design feature. When ambiguity comes into play, judgment becomes part of the equation. Administrative personnel, we believe, have a tendency to take conservative positions on matters of judgment. This is consistent with a role oriented culture, in which consistency in operations depends on standard operating procedures, not judgment. It is much to an agency's interest to have all or most decisions it makes based on what are called "programmed" decisions; programmed decisions are decisions that are based on a series of unequivocal "yes or no" binary choices. When decisions are programmed, administrative consistency is more assured and customers have less incentive to "shop" for a staff member who will be more amenable to suggested solutions to engineering problems that fall just outside the box.

The cost of retrofitting hospitals to comply with SB 1953 seems to us to have turned out to be much higher than most participants had anticipated. Certainly, the cost of replacing old hospitals with new ones was very expensive. As a consequence, both hospitals and their consulting engineers sought comparatively inexpensive ways to comply. As the engineers became more innovative, they increasingly challenged more conventional approaches to addressing problems, forcing more judgment into the decisions about what would meet program requirements.

Based on our interviews, it seems clear that judgment decisions gave rise to much of the conflict between engineers and OSHPD staff. Engineers tended to complain that staff members were too rigid and staff members sought to avoid errors by relying on how they read the regulations. Both of these perceptions are consistent with the values espoused by a role oriented culture. Those occupying each of the positions – regulator and petitioner – did what would be expected of them. As a consequence, some level of disagreement was inevitable.

7.3.5 *Implementation and Small "p" Politics*

When developing the program regulations that would operationalize the SB 1953 legislation, OSHPD was careful to seek the advice of hospital owners as well as active advocates for enhanced seismic safety in hospitals. It was the right thing to do. At the time, however, hospital owners found themselves in a difficult position. None of them could reasonably be expected to come out against seismic safety in hospitals, they had seen bills introduced in the legislature that were more Draconian than SB 1953, and, because they were so diverse, it was extremely unlikely that a unified position could be formulated that they might present to the framers of the regulations. Thus, for the most part, the owners went along with the regulations.

When they realized the full implications of the regulations, resistance to the program became evident and began to grow. Many, but not all, hospital owners viewed complying with SB 1953 regulations as an extraordinary burden coming at a time when their revenues were inadequate to cover their costs of doing business. Many of those owners and operators we interviewed saw the regulations as unnecessary and extraordinarily burdensome. Under those conditions, one would expect to see resistance to the regulations and pushback from hospital owners in various circumstances and that is what happened.

It became clear after the first few years following promulgation of the program regulations that hospital compliance with SB 1953 was going to be slow, extremely painful for some hospitals, and extraordinarily expensive. The legislature had failed to follow OSHPD's recommendation for financial assistance or relief in adopting the law. The legislature consistently failed to provide financial relief in the years that followed, even though it periodically provided relief to sets of hospitals in tightly defined circumstances. It is said that, to survive, organizations must pay attention to their customers' desires. One might say that hospitals were OSHPD's clients, but that would be a gross oversimplification. In reality, if they are to survive, organizations must be attentive to a set of constituencies, of which customers are only one. OSHPD's constituencies comprise other state agencies, including the Seismic Safety Council, that pursue their agenda through agencies like OSHPD. The organization must also be attentive to external interest groups, such as the Structural Engineers Association of California (SEAOC) which has, as part of its mission "to provide the public with structures of safe and dependable performance." SEAOC has seismic safety as a central focus of its activities and interests.

The hospitals that OSHPD regulates also comprise a constituency. For the hospitals, though, seismic safety is only one of a broad set of interests having to do with providing for service to physicians and patients, seismic safety for patients and staff, and ensuring organizational financial viability. In addition to these constituents, OSHPD must be attentive to leaders of the executive branch and legislators, particularly those who hold positions on committees with OSHPD oversight responsibilities. Often, if not most of the time, the constituencies have different agendas and different objectives with respect to OSHPD, and, even within agencies, while staff members will typically be in agreement with overall organizational goals, it is unlikely that all will share an equal commitment to one or another policies or practices. Complex and competing expectations from diverse constituents complicate decision making and action with agencies.

It is only within the above institutional context that one must examine both agency performance and generalized obstacles to implementing hazard mitigation policy. Experience suggests that bureaucracies, whether public or private, have a tendency to try to protect themselves from potential downside effects; organizations do not like to accept responsibility for things that go wrong. OSHPD was put into a position of having to find a viable balance among the demands of its constituent interests. The organization was committed to the goals inherent in SB 1953, but, taken together, hospital owners opposing the legislation and the rules could be expected to have considerable legislative clout. In light of those considerations, the literature suggests some possible agency behaviors.

Allison and Halperin (cited in Bardach 1977) suggest that the politics of the implementation process are highly defensive and that a great deal of energy goes into maneuvering to avoid responsibility, scrutiny, and blame. May and Williams (1986) observe that what passes for compliance activities often centers primarily on procedures rather than substantive issues unless care is taken to focus squarely and unequivocally on the primary objectives. We found OSHPD officials to be defensive, but did not see evidence of them attempting to avoid responsibility, scrutiny, or blame. To be sure, the legislation had intrinsic merit; earthquakes occur frequently in California, damage to hospitals from those events has been extensive, and, without enhanced seismic resistance, terrible scenarios can be readily envisaged for the future. Thus, it appears to us that most of the conflict was about when and how the enhanced seismic safety would be achieved and about undesirable side effects, but not about whether it should or would be achieved.

OSHPD was left largely on its own to defend the program, to cast it in the best light possible, and to devise means for ensuring that it would actually and ultimately achieve its goals. Clearly, no one in California government wanted to be put in a position of having to defend the program if a large number of hospitals failed to comply with various program deadlines. Periodically, the legislature enacted changes in the law to bring small clusters of hospitals into compliance with the law by granting them compliance extensions. The situation could have grown desperate had OSHPD not made a major change in policy. In retrospect, perhaps the single most critical event in the SB 1953 experience was that a very large number and proportion of California's hospital facilities were classified as SPC-1 at the beginning of 2001. The number was far larger than anyone had anticipated.

As engineers studied how to modify various old buildings to bring them into compliance, the individual and aggregate costs of retrofit began to be seen as untenable. Who would want to increase the seismic resistance of an old, largely obsolete building at extraordinary high cost with no prospects for recouping the investment? For all practical purposes the "rehab" program became a facility replacement program. Questions then arose as to whether sufficient engineering and construction capacity existed in the West to bring all the hospitals in compliance within the deadlines. OSHPD made what was clearly the most significant adaptation to the program when it was able to modify the methodology employed in the initial go-round of classifications. By adapting HAZUS to enable hospitals classified as SPC-1 in 2001 to be reevaluated and, if they passed the reevaluation, to be reclassified as SPC-2, the number of hospitals in need of virtually immediate repair, replacement, or closure was greatly reduced. Simultaneously, the number of hospital facilities in compliance was greatly increased. OSHPD was then able to proceed with a policy of fixing "the worst first."

The reclassifications resulting from the policy innovation greatly reduced the proportion of hospitals not in compliance with the law. No actual changes had been made to those facilities, but the new methodology reduced the number deemed to be in need of immediate action. Bardach (1977) observed that if there is sufficient leeway for the organization implementing the policy, the organization will act so as to maximize its organizational interest within constraints. OSHPD, along with others who supported the agency's overall goals with respect to hospital safety and the respect of its varied constituents, verified Bardach's observation and, in so doing, made a singularly critical change to improve the likelihood of program compliance by the regulated parties.

7.4 OSHPD'S Role

We concluded that the primary reasons for the difficulties associated with implementing SB 1953 had little to do with how OSHPD staff administered the program given the constraints placed upon it by other parts of the California government. The agency demonstrated professional and competent behavior under difficult circumstances, consistent with its mission, values, and culture. In the adoption of a modified HAZUS methodology, it demonstrated effective problem solving and program adaptation that went far beyond what one might expect from an administrative agency. This change was also consistent with its mission, values, and culture. OSHPD recognized the need to modify its approach and did so in a way that enabled it to meet the spirit and letter of SB 1953.

We do, though, find some obstacles to implementation with respect to OSHPD's role in formulating the SB 1953 policy. The California Seismic Safety Commission was the primary advocate for SB 1953 and, in fact, created draft legislation for the state legislature to consider. The legislature dropped some key provisions of the draft, including, perhaps most critically, a recommendation to provide financial assistance to hospitals to achieve seismic safety. The actual program regulations were drafted by the Hospital Building Safety Board. The Board is a part of OSHPD, having been established in the original Hospital Facilities Seismic Safety Act of 1973. It is charged with advising the Director of the Office of Statewide Health Planning and Development (OSHPD) on the administration of the Hospital Facilities Seismic Safety Act, and with acting as a board of appeals with regard to seismic safety and fire and life safety issues relating to hospital facilities. The Board includes nongovernmental practitioners appointed by OSHPD. The final regulations were the result considerable effort over a long time with lots of compromises and adjustments having been made through the process.

7.5 Looking for Answers Beyond the Usual Suspects

We've concluded that OSHPD's administration was not a determining factor in SB 1953s difficult road to implementation. What, then, are determining factors? The balance of Part II looks at several sources of barriers to implementation. In Part III, we look at how the regulated parties – hospital owners and operators – responded to the legislation and the program in terms of deciding whether to comply, how to comply, and when to comply. This is our attempt to address a long-overlooked part of regulatory policies. Regulatory policies do not work unless the targeted parties take action in response to them.

Part IV focuses on the extent to which two other clusters of variables affect implementation. The first has to do with how the problem is framed and with the policy and programs that are devised to bring about the desired effects. The second cluster has to do with the consequences of a dynamic institutional and socioeconomic context on implementation.

References

Alesch DJ, Petak WJ (2001) Overcoming obstacles to implementing earthquake hazard mitigation policies: stage 1 report. Multidisciplinary Center for Earthquake Engineering Research, Buffalo. Technical report MCEER-01-0004

Bardach (1977) What happens after a bill becomes law, MIT Press, Cambridge

Godschalk DR, Beatley T, Berke P, Brower DJ, Kaiser EJ, Bohl CC, Goebel RM (1999) Natural hazard mitigation: recasting disaster policy and planning. Island Press, Washington, DC

Harrison R (1979) Understanding your organization's character. Harv Bus Rev 57(5):119–128

Lipsky M (1971) Street level bureaucracy and the analysis of urban reform. Urban Aff Quart 6:391–409

May PJ, Williams W (1986) Disaster policy implementation: managing programs under shared governance. Plenum Press, New York

May PJ, Wood RS (2003) At the regulatory front lines: inspectors' enforcements styles and regulatory compliance. J Public Adm Res Theory 13(2):117–139

OSHPD (2011) Mission and values. http://www.oshpd.ca.gov/General_Info/Mission_and_Values.html

Pressman JL, Wildavsky A (1973) Implementation. University of California Press, Berkeley

Sabatier P, Mazmanian D (1979) The conditions of effective implementation: a guide to accomplishing policy objectives. Policy Anal 5:481–504

Schein EH (2010) Organizational culture and leadership, 4e. Jossey-Bass, San Francisco

Part III
Beyond the Usual Suspects: The Regulated Parties, Prerequisites to Action, and the Hazard Mitigation Investment Decision

This part examines the responses to the policy by the regulated parties – the owners and operators of acute care hospitals in California built before 1973 and judged not to be in compliance with State seismic safety provisions. Here, the authors examine what they call "the hazard mitigation investment decision" in the light of choices made by hospital owners about whether, when, and how to comply with the statutory mandates in SB 1953. They stress the importance of congruence between the policy and the inherent needs of the regulated parties.

Chapter 8
Organizational Responses: Introduction to Hazard Mitigation Investment Decision Making in Hospitals

8.1 Introduction

Hearing that we wanted to discuss how their hospital had or was planning to respond to SB 1953, two hospital administrators exchanged knowing glances. The one seated at the table chuckled quietly, while the other one, standing just inside the door of the conference room, declared, "Unfunded mandate" followed by, "What else would you like to know?"

Faced with the apparent objective reality of SB 1953, with its deadlines and potential consequences for non-compliance, California hospitals have had to contemplate a complex web of interdependent decisions. Contrary to what some SB 1953 advocates may have believed, the decisions that hospital administrators have had to make have not been simple ones. They have involved substantial capital commitments, extensive and not always well known opportunity costs, ongoing internal and external political maneuvering, consideration and reconsideration of decision fit with business strategy, establishing relationships with and evaluating the trustworthiness of architectural and engineering firms, and creativity in designing and implementing solutions that may not have been immediately apparent or appropriate. The decisions have not only been complex; they have had to be made again and again. As time has gone by, different players have joined the ranks of the decision makers and those charged with ensuring compliance with SB 1953 and the required regulations. Moreover, circumstances have regularly changed as amendments have been made to the law, as more information has become available, and as healthcare economics have continued to change. Traditional rational decision-making approaches have been found wanting, as "the problem" and possible solutions have been defined differently, depending on who was looking at them and when.

Decision complexity has conspired with each hospital's idiosyncratic characteristics to yield an array of decision choices. Many advocates and others uninvolved in the actual decision making may have believed that hospitals would simply comply with the legislation, since, after all, they had had at least 30 years to recognize

D.J. Alesch et al., *Natural Hazard Mitigation Policy: Implementation, Organizational Choice, and Contextual Dynamics*, Environmental Hazards,
DOI 10.1007/978-94-007-2235-4_8,

the need for and implement changes that would enhance seismic safety in their acute care facilities. In other words, advocates and others may have wanted to believe that SB 1953 and its enforcement would be sufficient by itself to ensure a shift in hospital decision-making attitudes and behaviors. The attitude seemed to be that, "while it might take some hospitals a few years to comply, eventually, all of them would do what was necessary." After all, if the hospitals couldn't see that seismic safety was a positive end in itself, surely the threat of not being allowed to operate as an acute care hospital would be enough to "encourage" proper behavior.

We were drawn into the study of SB 1953 one author at a time. One of the authors conducted a literature search on policy implementation in 1998 in part as a response to requests from OSHPD and others. Another of the authors later joined the effort and together, the authors began investigating SB 1953 and its implementation as a case study in policy implementation. A few years later the final author was invited to join the case study team and share her expertise on organizational decision making. This addition was seen as important because a fair number of acute care hospitals were either delaying or not planning to cooperate with the legislation as passed and the regulations as developed and enforced. In brief, these hospitals were not complying as expected. What would it take, we were asked, to gain their compliance? Further, what accounted for the array of their decision choices? Why had some hospitals decided to move forward with either retrofitting or rebuilding, while other hospitals were still in the process of weighing their options, thereby delaying their decision making? Why had still other hospitals decided unequivocally to neither retrofit nor rebuild their facilities?

A review of the decision-making literature provided some insight into possible answers to these and related questions. Likewise, conversations with OSHPD staff members and representative architects and structural engineers were also insightful. We had many conversations with interested parties who said things like, "Well, it's obvious that they ...," "they" being hospital decision makers. Still, we knew that the only people who could articulate for certain what "they" had decided to do and why were the actual decision makers, the hospital administrators. To that end, we decided to interview administrators from hospitals throughout California. Then, in order to assess the generalizability of what we had learned to states not having legislation akin to SB 1953, we decided to interview administrators from hospitals in Oregon and Washington, both susceptible to earthquakes. Finally, in order to assess the generalizability of what we had learned to states facing hazards other than earthquakes, we decided to interview administrators from hospitals in Louisiana and Mississippi, both susceptible to flooding and hurricanes.

Before embarking on our interviews, we defined the type of decision at the center of our research inquiry, the hazard mitigation investment decision. Such decisions have five key characteristics:

1. While they affect and are made by individuals, they are organizational decisions, not personal ones. Individuals such as members of the governing boards, CEOs, and CFOs are ultimately accountable for the decisions, but the decision's consequences accrue primarily to the organization.

2. Their purpose is to enhance the focal organization's resilience in response to hazardous events, especially extreme (low probability/high consequence) events. The events may be natural (e.g., earthquakes, hurricanes) or human-caused (e.g., terrorist attacks, pandemic flu). The likelihood of the event in question is understood to be rare, while the consequences of the event are understood to be negative and far-reaching. In all possible ways – material, physical, emotional, and intellectual – the potential consequences associated with extreme hazardous events are expected to affect individuals, organizations, their immediate communities, and beyond.
3. The costs (human, material, logistical, and financial) associated with such mitigation decisions are sufficiently high to warrant decision-making involvement and final approval from individuals at the highest level of the organization. Usually, the costs are sufficiently high to warrant budgeting for them over a multi-year timeframe. Likewise, the costs are sufficiently high to compel the diversion of resources away from other decision opportunities, such as acquisition of equipment.
4. The "solutions" tend to change over time, as engineers and other professionals learn more about hazards and building performance, and design new methods to mitigate against the negative consequences of various hazards.
5. The "solutions" seldom have the potential to add directly and positively to the organization's "bottom line." Instead, the mitigation falls squarely on the cost side of the standard "benefit-cost" analysis, with the solutions and possible benefits often invisible – literally – to all but those individuals whose business is hazard mitigation. While some people may believe that mitigation adds positive value to an organization's overall operations, it can be difficult to persuade decision makers to see benefits that may be observed over time (full cycle) vs. costs that are generated in the current fiscal year.

One outcome of our interview-based research is that we have come to believe that most organizations are not experienced at making decisions about investing resources to reduce the likely adverse consequences of extreme hazardous events. In lieu of direct experience, organizational decision makers tend to rely on their experience of making other kinds of decisions, on the experiences of professional colleagues or competitors in organizations facing the same or similar decisions, or on decision-making literature. Experience is often not a good teacher, especially when the experience has little in common with the current decision to be made. The bundle of characteristics that define extreme hazard mitigation investment decisions, described previously, is likely unique. For example, hazard mitigation investment decisions, especially those associated with extreme hazardous events, are often expensive, perhaps prohibitively so, and the "fixes" that are state-of-the-art today may be outdated before the current capital budgeting timeline expires. Further, the "fixes" may never be needed, as the probability of an extreme hazardous event occurring in close proximity to the individual hospital is relatively small and the probability that it will generate severe damage is even lower. Finally, by themselves, the "fixes" are unlikely to improve the organization's fiscal health.

After all, they're intended to forestall or minimize the negative consequences associated with a rare event, not to make the organization more attractive to stakeholders or more efficient.

In terms of relevant literature, organizational decision makers may turn to practitioner literature (e.g., publications distributed by professional associations) or academic literature (e.g., texts or journals read in college or available through the library). Traditional normative approaches to decision making, described in both the practitioner and academic literature, typically involve applying a univariate economic or financial analysis founded in the rational model of decision making. A normative benefit-cost analysis is typically favored for public sector organizations while investor-owned organizations are more likely to opt for return on investment or asset analyses. Regardless of the analysis used, the fundamental assumption underlying traditional decision making approaches is that cost is the primary criterion. Costs are believed to be objectively determinable and reliable, such that any knowledgeable individual assessing the decision making event would reach the same or nearly same conclusion as to the source and magnitude of relevant cost. Similarly, the benefits associated with the cost are assumed to be objectively determinable and reliable. Decision making, then, is a matter of "running the numbers" according to the appropriate algorithm, and acting in such a way that the costs of a given decision do not exceed its benefits.

In contrast to this approach, an approach that we have simplified greatly in our description in order to reveal some of its underlying assumptions, our research suggests that both private and public decision makers employ multiple criteria when making complex decisions, trading off among competing goals and, sometimes, among mutually exclusive objectives. How costs and benefits come to be perceived and accounted for is neither objectively determinable nor reliable. Certainly there have been attempts to increase the objectivity of the process that yields the numbers and of the process that evaluates the numbers. The insurance industry, for example, has expended considerable effort toward accurately calculating the probable maximum loss associated with various hazardous events (Woo 2002).

No matter how objective numbers may appear to be, decisions – including hazard mitigation decisions – are made by human beings whose capacity for rationality is limited. As March and Simon (1958) described so eloquently, human beings are boundedly rational. Our ability to define problems and generate and evaluate potential solutions is bounded by our intellectual capacity, which can consider only a relatively few options in the time available. Likewise, our personalities, values, and previous experiences serve to filter and distort so-called objective reality such that people in the same room facing the same situation at the same time will invariably describe it differently. Consequently, even something as seemingly objective as "benefit-cost analysis" can yield different outcomes thanks to the varying backgrounds, perceptions, and goals of those involved in the dialogue on benefits and costs. Costs that seem preeminent to one top manager may appear negligible to another. At the same time, both of these individuals are likely to say that "cost" is a major factor influencing their decision making.

Charged with the responsibility of leading their organizations into the future, hospital executives must take into account and balance the needs, expectations, and likely actions of multiple stakeholder groups. These stakeholders include owners, governing boards, physicians, nurses, other staff members, suppliers, the surrounding community, accrediting organizations, competitors, relevant government entities at the local, state, and federal levels, and, of course, patients. Each of these stakeholder groups may define "organizational effectiveness" differently, with some demanding maximum profits, some demanding low prices, some demanding higher wages, and others demanding organizational decisions that correspond to their vision of how hospital organizations should evaluate their priorities. Organizational politics are the inevitable result of competing priorities and goal incongruence. The end result? Decisions, especially decisions of magnitude, are not – and by definition, cannot be – optimized.

The research reported here aims at contributing to an understanding of how organizations actually make extreme hazard mitigation investment decisions. While our research is undertaken with SB 1953 and its regulations in mind, we avoid making the assumption that either laws or regulation alone dictate the form and outcome of organizational decision making. Instead, we view laws and their regulations as one set of possible predictors or constraining variables in a pool of potential predictor or constraining variables. As they do when considering costs and benefits, decision makers rely on their backgrounds, perceptions, and goals to ascertain the significance of laws and regulations and their likely effects on their organization's future. When it comes to organizational decision making around complex issues, perception *is* reality. Seemingly objective laws and regulations that stipulate apparently equal or at least equitable distribution of outcomes will be perceived differently by different organizations, all of which may choose to respond in completely different ways.

For example, although it is the objective case that SB 1953 has a nominal date certain for compliance, our interviews and data collected by Meade and Kulick (2007) suggest that, until recently, relatively few of the regulated organizations were convinced that compliance would be enforced by the published dates. Why? In part, they believed the adverse consequences of enforcing the mandate would be perceived as too great by the communities served. Ironically, SB 1953 and its enforcement appear to parallel the extreme natural hazards that SB 1953 seeks to compel mitigation against. Just as the consequence of an extreme natural hazard such as an earthquake can be severe, so too is the stated consequence of non-compliance with SB 1953 – the loss of licensure, which effectively makes it impossible for any affected organization to remain in business as an acute care hospital facility. Likewise, just as the likelihood of an extreme natural hazard is considered rare, by definition, so too is the perceived likelihood of an acute care hospital facility losing its license because it failed to comply with SB 1953 by the stated deadline. Hence, for many organizational decision makers, the perception of benefit-cost does not match the "objective reality" of benefit-cost described in the regulations. For people who are accustomed to making decisions under conditions of risk, neither the "odds" of a devastating earthquake nor the "odds" of licensure loss may be seen as sufficiently great to warrant action.

Perception drives behavior. Hence, in the first decade following the development of the regulations, relatively few hospital organizations committed resources to compliance with the more costly and less credible elements of the regulations. Now that the regulations have been revised in accord with HAZUS, modifying the extent of the problem to be addressed, we see changing perceptions and, therefore, changing behaviors.

While SB 1953 was the "hook" that initially attracted us to this research, our purpose is not limited to examining whether, why, and how organizations choose to comply with SB 1953. Instead, our purpose goes beyond understanding organizational response to legislative mandate to consider whether, why, and how organizations make all hazard mitigation investment decisions, regardless of their genesis. SB 1953 serves as the lens through which we examine this broader issue. If "objective" regulation with deleterious consequences for non-compliance can't compel desired behavior, then what will? We believe that the answers to this question will enable us to better understand whether, why, and how organizations make extreme hazard mitigation investment decisions. Consequently, we believe that our behavioral research will add to the authenticity of existing normative models for making these complex and difficult decisions, and increase their potential for enabling good decisions.

8.2 Overview of Our Theoretical Framework

As described earlier, and as we learned through our interviews, the process of hazard mitigation investment decision making is complicated, and its outcomes are difficult to predict. First, hazard mitigation investments typically consume substantial resources, especially when the mitigation involves large building construction or alteration. Money spent on hazard mitigation is money not spent on other projects or activities. The greater the amount of money spent on hazard mitigation, the greater the amount not available for other projects, and the larger the potential opportunity cost associated with the hazard mitigation expenditure.

Second, the individuals involved in making hazard mitigation investment decisions are often not experts in hazard mitigation, but are experts instead in managing their particular enterprise. To that end, key decision makers find themselves having to rely on the professional judgment of individuals whom they may not fully trust or understand to give them options with respect to hazard mitigation investments. In situations of uncertainty like this, decision makers may not be confident that they know the right questions to ask, or when, or even how to interpret the responses to the questions. In addition to top managers lacking expertise in the area of hazard mitigation, it's also important to recognize that hazard mitigation is a relatively small piece of the ever-changing puzzle that these key individuals must continually manage.

Third, like so many other things, hazard mitigation is an evolving discipline, such that today's "state-of-the-art" may be outdated in short order, perhaps before a given hazard mitigation is completed (e.g., before an existing building is fully retrofitted or a new building is built). New, more effective, and sometimes less expensive options for hazard mitigation are routinely developed as academics discover new solutions and practitioners find efficient means for implementation. The costs and timeline associated with retrofitting a large and complex building, such as an acute care hospital building, are difficult to specify with any degree of accuracy, because unanticipated problems tend to appear with shocking regularity. Where building plans indicate the presence of piping and electrical systems, actual demolition reveals something else altogether. Relatively few engineering firms specialize in retrofitting complex structures, reducing the likelihood that a given firm will have the expertise necessary to develop highly accurate cost and timeline estimates. No one, including the affected engineering firms, is satisfied with this reality. Several of those we interviewed said they would do anything to avoid retrofitting their structures, because they "just knew" that doing so would unleash a Pandora's box of unexpected problems and unmanageable costs and delays.

Finally, the hazard mitigation investment decision making process tends to be non-linear, as participants find themselves returning to various decision points over time. Whether and when these decision points are revisited depends on various internal and external conditions and causes. For example, change in the composition of the organization's top management team may cause the organization to revisit completely its decision-making process and intermediate decisions. Likewise, change in the cost of materials might make do-able a formerly impossible solution, or vice versa. In fact, there may be multiple paths to a "fix," with none clearly emerging as the winner.

Our understanding of the hazard mitigation investment decision-making process and its outcomes has developed considerably over the course of our research. Initially, we assumed that the decision-making process could be understood using a typical research approach in which we would specify a dependent variable and then hypothesize its relationship to several explanatory variables. To that end, and presuming a linear and fairly uncomplicated decision-making process, we began our research by selecting "compliance with the statutory requirements" as our dependent variable. The "statutory requirement" of interest was SB 1953. The goal was to determine what predicted organizational compliance with SB 1953. We reasoned that if we could determine the key predictors of compliance, then individuals and organizations (e.g., advocates) hoping to increase and ease compliance could focus their time and efforts appropriately.

Unfortunately, interviews with healthcare executives suggested that our dependent variable was not as simply defined as we had believed. Instead, it was a **moving target**. The choice of whether to comply with SB 1953 and, if so, how, was rarely made by the authorized organizational decision makers once and for all or even early in the period allowed for compliance. The decision of whether and how to comply was made in the healthcare organizations we interviewed over a multi-year period. Several organizations interviewed were waiting to make their "final" decisions. Some that made decisions earlier changed them later. As deadlines approached, very few had committed resources to a decision. Even fewer had a specific timeline for completion. Most seemed to be in "limbo," not wanting to ignore the regulations, but not sure whether and how to proceed, despite considerable internal dialogue and external consultation, along with pressure and vagaries in direction from the regulatory body – OSHPD.

Many pointed to numerous versions of in-house plans that had been generated and dismissed over the course of many years. "When we thought this what was we needed to do, and these were the resources we had available, we planned to do this. Then, everything changed, and those plans were shelved." During more than one interview, we were invited to examine the piles of rejected "solutions."

Recognizing that organizations thought more broadly and more often about the SB 1953 decision than we initially believed, we decided to broaden our focus beyond "compliance with SB 1953" to address all "extreme hazard mitigation investment decisions." We also accepted that our initial assumption that the compliance decision was a one-time decision – e.g., "we decided in late October, 2005 to move forward and we have done so" – was fundamentally flawed and did not capture the reality of most organizations' decision making.

This prompted us to ask several questions central to understanding the case of SB 1953 and identifying its broader implications. Why was the decision about whether, why, and how to comply with SB 1953 so complicated? Why did organizational decision makers choose to revisit and revise their decision as often as they did? What factors, besides regulation, did organizational decision makers consider when making extreme hazard mitigation investment decisions?

What appears to have happened and to be happening is that many of the organizational decision makers we interviewed, after analyzing the likely costs of retrofitting their buildings against the earthquake threat, found the costs to be exceptionally and prohibitively high. The high costs stem from three sources: (1) the *actual* costs of strengthening the building, (2) the *logistical* costs associated with interrupting acute care operations (and sequentially shifting the location of operations to accommodate reconstruction), and (3) the *supplemental* and often high costs that arise from complying with other costly building regulations that are triggered when major changes are made to buildings.

The high costs were deemed especially problematic in that retrofitting existing buildings often meant expending significant resources only to end up with a facility that may have been outdated in terms of its ability to deliver requested services. Old bed towers, for example, tend to feature rooms intended for more than one patient. For at least the past two decades, hospitals have seen a steady increase in the number of patients wanting private rooms. Old surgical centers tend to be inadequate in terms of electrical and computer capability. High-end surgeries involve both robotics and computers. For many hospitals, the bottom line was relatively simple: They would spend a great deal of money and have little to show for it, at least from the perspective of key stakeholders such as patients and surgical staff.

If benefits are believed to outweigh costs, and organizations have access to needed resources, then the organization may proceed with a given decision. But no amount of likely or perceived benefit can move a decision if resources are inadequate, unavailable, or prohibitively costly to acquire. The problem of high costs was exacerbated for most healthcare organizations because about 85% of California acute care hospitals were losing money – hemorrhaging, really – in the late 1990s when SB 1953 came into force. Many are still losing money, primarily because of having to shift from a cost-plus financial basis to a highly competitive business in which HMO and Medicare reimbursements do not always cover the costs of treatment. Thus, the SB 1953 compliance requirement was seen by most hospitals as simply one more consideration in corporate strategic business planning focused on getting and remaining solvent. As extreme hazard mitigation investment decisions go, the decision to comply with SB 1953 was going to cost affected organizations a potentially excessive amount given the low perceived likelihood of devastating seismic activity and the uncertain-at-best benefits to the organization's bottom line, reputation, and ability to fulfill its organizational mission.

As their financial circumstances have changed in the time since the law was enacted and the administrative regulations were produced, California's healthcare organizations have explored various means for adapting their businesses to an increasingly hostile external environment while, at the same time, complying with SB 1953s seismic safety rules. Competition for financial resources, human resources, information resources, and physical resources has escalated. The shift in environmental munificence (Dess and Beard 1984) for many key resources from apparently abundant to increasingly scarce has intensified the amount of environmental uncertainty facing California's hospitals, and altered the type and complexity of all organizational decisions, including those dealing with SB 1953.

For most of the hospital organizations studied, the decision making process has been nonlinear and episodic. Decision making criteria have changed as circumstances have changed for both the industry and its individual healthcare organizations. Options that may have been considered outlandish or cost-prohibitive in one year may find favor in another year because circumstances have changed and, with them, what is possible or impossible. Decisions associated with SB 1953 have had to be made alongside complex decisions about staffing, equipment, real estate, services offered, community engagement, competitive strategy, and others.

Thus, measuring "whether organizations comply" has become "the extent to which organizations comply" and "how they choose to comply." In some cases, the answer for each organization has been known to change over a period of months. Since virtually all of the affected organizations face proportionally high costs coupled with relatively low benefits for complying with SB 1953, we asked, "**What accounts for the myriad decisions made over time** (e.g., to retrofit existing facilities, to build new facilities, to close existing facilities and not build new ones, to change from an acute care to a different kind of facility)"? This has become our driving research question.

The research challenge is further complicated because there is uncertainty, even disbelief, among the regulated as to whether the prospective sanction, i.e., loss of license, is a viable threat. As is the general case with extreme hazard mitigation investment decisions, the potential outcome is considered rare. Some hospital executives have argued that the State of California will not close hospitals in underserved areas that cannot or choose not to comply with SB 1953. After all, doing so would simply ensure that those acute care hospitals would be closed both before **and** after an earthquake disaster. Such a counterproductive move strikes some as untenable. Thus, the threat may not serve its intended purpose of compelling compliance because key decision makers do not perceive that the threat will be enforced.

As they say, "If the idea behind SB 1953 is to ensure uninterrupted access to acute care throughout the State, why would anyone choose to close acute care hospitals?" Threatened punishment must be believable to be effective (Skinner 1974). People respond to salient rewards and punishments, not to those they deem unlikely or irrelevant to their ongoing behavior.

Similarly, it appears that many California hospital executives do not believe in earthquakes. This statement is not intended to be amusing. Instead, it is meant to reflect our observation that many top hospital executives do not believe that a devastating earthquake will affect their hospital facility any time in the relevant future. So, while they may believe in earthquakes and their negative consequences in general, they do not believe in them in specific, at least not enough to be frightened or compelled into action. The devastating earthquake described by seismic safety advocates and others is possible, but not probable, at least as far as many top decision makers are concerned. Consequently, neither the threat of non-licensure nor the threat of earthquake is sufficient to alter behavior. Neither threat is perceived to be credible.

We are not arguing that earthquakes are not believable. Nor are we arguing that organizational decision makers should ignore the potentially deleterious consequences of a destructive earthquake. We believe in earthquakes, and we believe that they are a threat to life safety, business continuation, and society's quality of life. We believe that organizations have a moral obligation to prepare for and address likely hazards.

We also believe that we cannot and should not impose our beliefs on the people and decisions that we are trying to understand. Hence, we view our job as describing what we have observed, while trying to minimize our judgment of such. In the end, we believe this approach will enable better decision making on the part of organizational decision makers and on the part of extreme hazard safety advocates.

In brief, we have discovered that key decision makers' perceptions of the problem, potential solutions, and likely consequences are central to understanding their decisions and the process used to reach those decisions. We have learned that looking at SB 1953 as an objectively-defined law and associated regulations with an objectively-defined consequence for failure to comply is counterproductive to our accurately understanding hospital decision makers' decision making processes and chosen outcomes. Consistent with cognitive appraisal theory (Lazarus and Folkman 1984), we believe it is decision makers' **perceptions** that matter, perceptions that depend on their individual and their hospital's circumstances and context. Thus, we should not expect to observe undifferentiated responses to and engagement with the extreme hazard mitigation investment decision.

Consequently, we have developed our theoretical framework in line with Weick's (1995, 2001) description of sensemaking in organizations. Our goal is to describe the process and outcomes associated with hazard mitigation investment decisions from the perspective of those involved in making these decisions. We want to understand hazard mitigation investment decision making as it is understood by those who do it. What we have learned thus far about hazard mitigation investment decisions suggests that any search for and attempt to describe a linear and rational formal decision making process will prove futile. Indeed, we think that the actual non-linear and quasi-rational decision making process may be far more interesting to ponder, and is certainly more useful to document.

Several key elements characterize sensemaking (Weick 1995). First, sensemaking involves seeing through the eye of the beholder. To understand how and why a particular decision was made, one needs access to the thinking and perceptions of key decision makers. Second, sensemaking is a social process based on retrospective consideration of historical thinking and action. Third, sensemaking is ongoing, a never-ending process in which past actions are considered, reconsidered, and considered anew. Whereas "decision making" implies a process that yields a finite conclusion, sensemaking implies a process that yields a tentative conclusion, one that is subject to continued examination and refinement. Fourth, sensemaking derives from a relatively small set of cues extracted from myriad cues in the environment. We are not able to evaluate all relevant points of data. Instead, we ponder that which is immediate, that which reminds us of something we already know, that which supports our existing perceptions. Finally, sensemaking is driven by plausibility, not accuracy. Once people find what they construe to be an answer to a question, they stop looking for additional, possibly more correct, answers. As described by Weick (2001, p. 96),

> Sensemaking generates understanding that is provisional, plausible, subject to revision, swift, directed toward continuation of interrupted activity, ready-to-hand, tentative, infused with ignorance, and sufficient for current purposes. ... Sensemaking starts out as momentary, expedient understanding. But the sense thus created often lingers and gets stored as if it were the product of a far more deliberate, intentional analysis.

In general, we have used the sensemaking "lens" to help us understand the hazard mitigation investment decision making process as it occurs in organizations, or at least as it is believed to occur in organizations from the perspective of key organizational decision makers. In particular, we have used this lens to help us understand the extreme hazard mitigation investment decision-making process used in California hospital organizations facing SB 1953. While we rely on the sensemaking lens to guide our thinking about extreme hazard mitigation investment decision making, we continue to use the more commonly-heard phrase "decision making," since the phrase "sensemaking" is neither well-understood nor typically used.

Our theoretical framework has two major components. In the first component, we review (Petak and Alesch 2004) five organizational prerequisites for adoption and implementation of hazard mitigation measures. Building on the influential work of March and Olsen (1973), the five prerequisites include: awareness of the issue, belief that action is possible, belief that now is the right time to act, existence of an acceptable solution, and capacity to act. The five prerequisites set the stage for organizational action, and are fundamental to our understanding the process and outcomes associated with hazard mitigation investment decisions in organizations.

While the prerequisites to action serve as the foundation of our thinking, their purpose is more descriptive with respect to generalized organizational process than predictive with respect to specific organizations and their actual process and outcomes. As stated by Petak and Alesch (2004, pp. 128–129),

> ... While all the organizations we studied engaged in the same general process, individual processes varied in detail and emphasis. Moreover, virtually none of the organizations engaged

in a strictly linear approach to solving the problem. Most organizations addressed it iteratively, circling back to earlier assumptions, building in new information and new perceptions, and rethinking options, discarding some, fleshing others out, and searching for new ones.

If the prerequisites to action are general in nature, and if actual decision-making process and outcomes vary by organization, then what accounts for these differences? We attempt to address this essential question in the second component of our theoretical narrative, where we present critical categories of factors that we believe influence whether, why, and how organizations make extreme hazard mitigation investment decisions. We describe each category from a theoretical perspective, drawing on relevant academic literature. Then, we augment our description of each category with examples drawn from our qualitative research. As expected, the examples capture decision making by California hospitals facing the decision to comply with SB 1953. Perhaps unexpectedly, the examples also capture decision making by hospitals facing seismic threats in Oregon and Washington, and by hospitals facing hurricane threats in Louisiana and Mississippi. In this way, our examples illustrate the impact of the critical categories beyond the environment of SB 1953.

The second part of our theoretical framework incorporates several critical categories of factors believed influential in the extreme hazard mitigation investment decision-making process. The factors are drawn from literature on upper-echelons, as initially described by Hambrick and Mason (1984), from Porter's (1980) work on organizational strategy, and from the literature on transaction cost economics (e.g., Williamson 1975). The factors are also drawn from the literature on institutional isomorphism (e.g., DiMaggio and Powell 1983), and on regulatory relationships (e.g., Rothwell 1992).

First, Hambrick and Mason (1984) make a strong case that the characteristics of those occupying an organization's upper-echelons condition the organization's decision-making process and outcomes. Thus, the functional background, experience, perceptions, and so on of the individual members of the organization's top management team are expected to affect how the organization proceeds when faced with making hazard mitigation investment decisions.

Second, organizational strategy is expected to influence hazard mitigation investment decision making. As described by Porter (1980), the particular generic business-level strategy adopted by an organization consequently affects or is expected to affect decisions around resource allocation. Organizations tend to align with one of three generic strategies: differentiation, low cost leadership, or focus. Each of these strategies makes different assumptions about the market to be served and the approach to serving the chosen market. Whether and to what extent an organization decides to invest in hazard mitigation would seem to depend in part on whether the organization's decision makers believe that the investment would align with the organization's chosen strategy.

Third, whether and how an organization decides to invest in hazard mitigation around extreme events would seem to depend in part on the economic feasibility of doing so. Drawing on Williamson's (1975) work, we suggest that whether and how an organization decides to invest in hazard mitigation around extreme events depends in part on whether the organization believes that such investments will yield a profitable return. Faced with an array of possibilities for using available capital, which investments are likely to produce the greatest return? Such is one of the themes associated with transaction cost economic theory.

Fourth, institutional theory provides insight into the external and internal forces that might be expected to both facilitate and hinder hazard mitigation investment decision making. Looking at DiMaggio and Powell's (1983) work, for example, we can see that there are forces external to the organization that compel it to behave like other, similar organizations and that yield similar organizational outcomes. Specifically, DiMaggio and Powell (1983) assert that there are coercive, normative, and mimetic forces. These forces emanate from the legal or regulatory context, shared professional values, and competition. Internally, there are forces that compel organizations to behave in certain ways, such as the organization's established structure and culture and formally sanctioned decision-making process.

Finally, the nature of the regulatory relationship is expected to influence the process and outcome of organizational decision making around hazard mitigation. In looking at the particular case of innovation, for example, Rothwell (1992) identified several characteristics of the regulatory relationship expected to influence decision making. Those characteristics included degree or intensity of the regulation, competence of the regulators, and collaboration in developing regulations.

References

Dess GG, Beard DW (1984) Dimensions of organizational task environments. Adm Sci Q 29:52–73

DiMaggio PJ, Powell WW (1983) The iron cage revisited: institutional isomorphism and collective rationality in the organizational field. Am Social Rev 48:147–160

Hambrick D, Mason P (1984) Upper echelons: the organization as a reflection of its top managers. Acad Manage Rev 9:193–206

Lazarus RS, Folkman S (1984) Stress, appraisal, and coping. Springer, New York

March JG, Olsen JP (1973) Ambiguity and choice in organizations. Universitetsforlaget, Bergen

March JG, Simon HA (1958) Organizations. Wiley, New York

Meade C, Kulick J (2007) SB 1953 and the challenge of hospital seismic safety in California. California HealthCare Foundation, Oakland

Petak WJ, Alesch DJ (2004) Organizational decision making with respect to extreme events: healthcare organizations respond to California's SB 1953. In research progress and accomplishments: 2003–2004 (MCEER-04-SP01). University of Buffalo, State University of New York, Multidisciplinary Center for Earthquake Engineering Research, Buffalo, May 2004

Porter M (1980) Competitive strategy. Free Press, New York

Rothwell R (1992) Industrial innovation and government environmental regulation: some lessons from the past. Technovation 12(7):447–458

Skinner BF (1974) About behaviorism. Vintage, New York

Weick KE (1995) Sensemaking in organizations. Sage, Thousand Oaks

Weick KE (2001) Making sense of the organization. Blackwell Publishing, Alden

Williamson OE (1975) Markets and hierarchies: analysis and antitrust implications. Free Press, New York

Woo G (2002) Natural catastrophe probable maximum loss. Br Actuar J 8:943–959, Part V

Chapter 9
Prerequisites to Organizational Action

9.1 Introduction

Much of the public policy literature on implementation of hazard mitigation or risk reduction measures focuses on why implementation is ineffective or inadequate in one or another settings. Clearly, it is important to understand the obstacles to implementation of hazard mitigation measures in order to better understand how to increase the probability of implementation. Likewise, it is important to focus on the other side of the equation; that is, under what conditions will organizations choose to invest in hazard mitigation measures? In other words, what facilitates the implementation of, or investment in, hazard mitigation measures?

Petak and Alesch's (2004) work on the prerequisites to organizational action was inspired by March and Olsen's (1973) garbage can model of organizational decision making. That model suggests that decisions are not made, nor are actions taken, unless four independent streams come together simultaneously. The four streams consist of a problem (about which there is general agreement within the organization), a solution to the problem (which is credible for a critical mass of actors within the organization), space on the organizational agenda, and one or more persistent advocates for matching the available solution with the existing problem. Based on their preliminary understanding of hospitals' response to SB 1953, Petak and Alesch (2004) identified five fundamental organizational prerequisites for adoption and implementation of extreme hazard mitigation measures. We discuss each in turn (Fig. 9.1).

9.2 The Organization Is Aware of the Issue

The first prerequisite for implementation of extreme hazard mitigation measures is that the organization's key decision makers must **perceive that the organization is at risk from an extreme hazard**, such as earthquakes. This is similar to March and Olsen's (1973) problem prerequisite.

D.J. Alesch et al., *Natural Hazard Mitigation Policy: Implementation, Organizational Choice, and Contextual Dynamics*, Environmental Hazards, DOI 10.1007/978-94-007-2235-4_9,

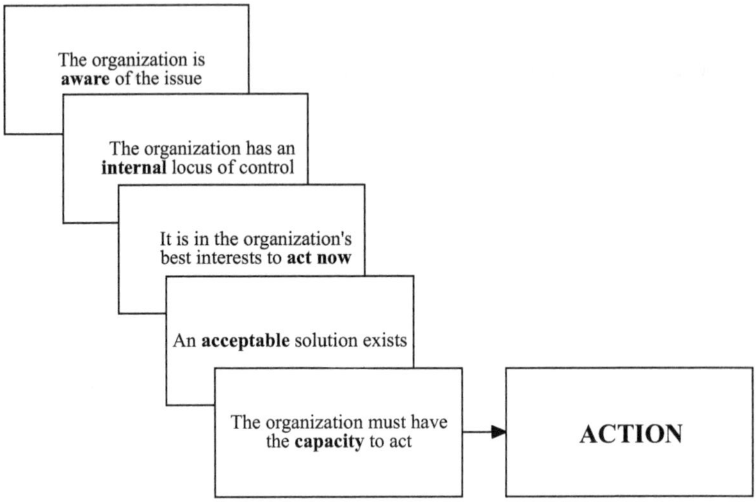

Fig. 9.1 Prerequisites to organizational action (Source: Petak and Alesch (2004))

Problems exist for organizations only when there is a difference between what the organization's key decision makers (i.e., top-level managers or Board of Directors, representing owners) desire and expect for the organization, and their perception of the state of affairs in which they find or expect to find the organization. In brief, there needs to be a disparity or gap between the decision makers' desired and perceived reality. Consequently, we would not expect an organization to invest in extreme hazard mitigation unless key organizational decision makers are dissatisfied with their perceptions of the current or projected situation and decide that a problem exists.

Traditional models of risk assessment look at the hazard, exposure, vulnerability, and probable maximum losses from events of various magnitudes (Woo 2002). For example, for organizations to perceive themselves as having an "earthquake problem," a critical mass of key decision makers must believe that a credible earthquake hazard exists, that it is likely to occur within a relevant time frame, and that, should it occur, the organization would suffer more than trivial losses.

In considering the specific case of seismic mitigation, while it may be difficult for seismic scientists to accept that there are individuals and organizations in California who **do not believe** in the inevitability of damaging earthquakes and the subsequent negative consequences for life and property, proof that such individuals exist is presented every time someone is quoted in the news media saying something like, "I never thought that my house (business, school, church, etc.) would be affected." While those in the scientific community may tend to believe that these individuals and organizations *underestimate* the risks to which they are exposed, many of these individuals and organizations believe that the scientific community *overestimates* the risks. Every week, month, and year that goes by without a damaging earthquake seems to bolster the case of the non-scientific community, at least from its perspective. Belief in something depends on experience with that something, or on trust in another person's experience or statement of fact. Data presented as "facts" are often debatable. And scientists are often questioned about their theories as if scientific "facts" were no more than one group's beliefs. (Witness the debate around climate change, and the perceptions of many people that it isn't real, despite scientific evidence to the contrary.) Knowing that a geographic area is prone to a particular extreme hazard does not, in and of itself, persuade that such an event is inevitable. In this case, seeing is believing.

An excellent example of the relevance of perception and the rejection of scientific "fact" was shared with one of the authors while she was doing field research in Christchurch, New Zealand, after its September 4, 2010 earthquake. While chatting with a local New Zealander about the earthquake and the likelihood of future earthquakes, the local commented that he didn't think much of scientific projections and probabilities because he believed in biblical accounts of time rather than scientific accounts of the same. Clearly, individual perceptions are influenced by myriad factors, of which scientific "fact" is only one.

At the same time, and perhaps paradoxically, many members of the general public, including hospital executives, want to believe that building codes have been designed to address not only life safety, but immediate business and community continuity. In other words, they put tremendous faith in the ability of code designers and enforcers to ensure that people will survive and buildings will stand in the aftermath of an earthquake. Building design codes are not within the intellectual or interest domain of the average person, and so average people empower those with professional expertise to make the right decision on their behalf. An example of this willingness to entrust others with decision-making authority and consequent accountability may be found in stories of New Orleanians in the wake of Hurricane Katrina, who believed that the levees built and maintained by the Army Corps of Engineers would protect their homes. This belief in the Corps' ability to make appropriate professional decisions about controlling the natural environment persisted, despite the fact that these same "non-engineer" homeowners could see for themselves that the water in the canals was higher than their properties. In this case, seeing was not believing. People wanted to believe that the professionals must know something not revealed by their own eyes.

Why is it that seeing is believing in one case, but seeing is not believing in another? Probably many variables. We suggest that perceived cost (what it is, who bears it) is one critical variable. In the case of whether to believe scientists who say that a devastating earthquake is imminent and that individuals and organizations should take appropriate precautions, the scientists are not offering to bear the costs associated with hazard mitigation. In brief, the average person is likely to respond with something like, "It's easy for you to say I should do X, since you're not paying for it." In the case of whether to believe that design codes are appropriate (or, that levees will withstand rushing water), average people do not perceive that they are bearing the costs of development or enforcement, because the costs are often "hidden" from the average person's view. We're not suggesting that the costs are intentionally hidden (we don't think they are), but rather that the average person does not perceive them. The cost of enforcing building codes are borne first by contractors and eventually passed on to end-users. Likewise, the cost of maintaining levee systems are borne first by the relevant government agency and eventually paid for by taxpayers. In brief, we think it's relatively easy for the average person to have faith in code designers and similar experts and to delegate authority and responsibility to them because they don't have to write them a check for services rendered. Or, the check they write isn't associated with an itemized list of costs.

A key element in risk perception and problem definition has to do with timing. No one knows enough to predict earthquakes in anything but a geologic time frame. In general, individuals who are not members of the seismic scientific community, including top managers of hospital organizations, have a hard time understanding return periods and understanding that no one knows the location of all potential earthquake faults. Even if one accepts the inevitability of a damaging earthquake, if the threat is not perceived as likely within one's relevant time frame, the salience of the risk is minimal because the individual or organization does not perceive a risk that justifies action.

More often than we care to admit, we have heard people say things like, "Well, they say that the last big earthquake was a 100-year earthquake, and that was 15 years ago. So, we don't need to worry for another 85 years." Few people, it seems, understand probabilistic statistics. They are willing to gamble, even when they don't fully understand the probability of winning or losing, because they don't understand that hazardous events are usually independent of one another. In other words, they don't understand that this year's extreme hazardous event most likely has no impact on whether next year will bring another extreme event. Common logic dictates that if a slot machine hasn't paid out in a while, it's bound to pay out soon. Likewise, if it has recently paid out, it probably won't pay out for a while. Common logic presumes that events are dependent. Actual experience suggests otherwise.

Finally, it is not enough for individuals and organizations to believe in the likelihood of a damaging earthquake. If we expect organizations to take action to protect themselves, they have to understand their exposure, vulnerability, and the likelihood of adverse consequences when the event occurs. They must expect to incur meaningful losses. Knowing that there will be some amount of damage from an earthquake is not the same as expecting significant and adverse consequences from it. Again, it seems that most people prefer to assume the positive, that is, they assume that their losses will be minimal. Often, they base these assumptions on irrelevant experiential data (e.g., "The few hospitals that have experienced serious earthquakes in the last 20 years have not been seriously damaged" – never mind that the hospitals referenced were built recently and are more seismically resilient than their facilities).

9.3 The Organization Has an Internal Locus of Control

The second prerequisite for implementation of extreme hazard mitigation measures is that the organization must **believe that actions taken to mitigate extreme hazard risks will be effective**. Key decision makers must trust that their hazard mitigation investments will yield desired outcomes: In the specific case of earthquakes, hospitals must remain standing after earthquakes, such that the safety of patients and staff members is protected and such that key assets (e.g., medical equipment, HVAC units) remain operational. This second prerequisite represents an addition to March and Olsen's (1973) model.

Locus of control is a well-known personality trait associated with individuals' generalized belief in internal versus external control of reinforcement (Rotter 1966). An organization's top management team may be understood to possess "team" locus of control (Boone et al. 2005), such that a team comprising predominantly individuals with an internal locus of control is likely to develop a collective sense of potency (Shea and Guzzo 1987). In contrast, a team comprising predominantly individuals with an external locus of control is not likely do so. Top management teams with a collective sense of potency will believe that they can influence positively their own processes and outcomes, such as the quality of their decision-making process and its outcomes. As described by Shea and Guzzo (1987, p. 26), a collective sense of potency is a key group-level factor that determines "real-world, real-time group effectiveness." A self-reinforcing loop is created as high potency teams seek sometimes negative information to enhance the effectiveness of their decision making, which in turn enhances their decision making, which in turn enhances their collective potency, and so on.

In general, organizations with an internal locus of control (i.e., organizations led by top management teams with a collective internal locus of control) are likely to believe that they can exert some measure of control over extreme hazards by means of implementing appropriate risk reduction measures. Key decision makers in these organizations believe that practical steps exist to reduce the risks associated with extreme hazard events. They also believe that these steps are congruent with the nature and extent of the problem and with the organization's best interests. In contrast, organizations with an external locus of control may believe that no amount of risk reduction will prove sufficient in the face of an extreme hazard, such as a damaging earthquake or a hurricane followed by debilitating flooding. Key decision makers in these organizations may adopt an almost fatalistic posture, "No matter what we do, we cannot protect our facility, equipment, and stakeholders from the harm associated with an extreme hazard." Similarly, they may say such things as, "We can't mitigate against a disaster we haven't experienced." Whether a hospital organization has an internal vs. external locus of control with respect to extreme hazard mitigation likely depends on its relationship with reputable structural engineering firms, the trust placed in its own facilities management personnel, and the quantity and quality of extreme hazardous event experience possessed by the top management team. The more experience with hazards, the more likely that top managers will be able to accurately assess their facilities' vulnerabilities.

9.4 It Is in the Organization's Best Interests to Act Now

March and Simon (1958) created a simple, yet robust model of organizational decision making to explain a set of choices. The model suggests that key decision makers in organizations seek alternatives to what they are doing when they are dissatisfied with the way things are going. They keep searching as long as they believe there is a reasonable solution that can be found for less than the cost of the search, or when they find an acceptable alternative, or when they come to believe they cannot do better than they are doing now. Organizations take action when a critical mass of key decision makers believes either they or **the organization will be better off taking the action now rather than either deferring the action or not taking it at all**.

Alesch and Petak (1986) relate the story of an 85-year-old woman who testified before a Committee of the Los Angeles City Council that was deliberating what was to become of the city's unreinforced masonry building retrofit ordinance. "Let me understand this," she said. "You want to increase my rent by $50 a month for sure, forcing me to choose between medicine and food, because there *might* be an earthquake that *might* damage my building and I *might* be injured. Are you gentlemen playing with all your marbles?"

This story illustrates a critical issue. Individuals and organizations have more ways to use resources than they have resources. When given a choice of how to use those resources, most individuals and organizations aspire to make apparently rational choices. Most organizations, for example, will consider carefully the marginal utility of a dollar spent to reduce risk compared with the marginal utility of a dollar spent elsewhere. Then, given their preferences and their perception of the probable payoffs from alternative courses of action to realize those preferences, they will spend appropriately, for the most part. Of course, some people and organizations are better than others are at making good choices. This also assumes that the marginal costs and revenues or payoffs are known or are knowable, that the values of all decision makers are aligned, and that decision makers have the experience and expertise to accurately weigh and assess the available data.

Implementation problems for public policy are likely when governments enact policies dictating that some specific hazard mitigation measures be taken by a class of organizations regardless of the calculus of those individual organizations concerning risk and potential payoff. As suggested by the story of the 85-year-old woman, organizations will resist implementing those policies if their subjective estimates of the risks and payoffs and of relative priorities do not coincide with those of the governmental policy makers and advocates.

The individual organization's economic analysis of the financial benefits of reducing risks by employing one or another hazard mitigation technology is important, but only part of the story. In general, organizations do not implement policies unless those policies pass several tests. Not only must a proposed hazard mitigation policy make financial sense today, it must also be congruent with the organization's current goals (Vroom 1964), and align with the organization's priorities. Organizations will evaluate the costs associated with a given hazard mitigation measure, and assess the likelihood that the costs will increase or decrease in a given time frame. Likewise, organizations will consider the potential contribution or benefit of a given hazard mitigation measure to the organization's current vs. future goals. Such **benefit-cost ratio analysis** will be critical to choosing from an array of hazard mitigation measures. Of course, the specific array of goals and priorities will be unique to a given organization. Consequently, a hazard mitigation practice that makes sense this year for one organization may not make sense for another until next year, even later, or never.

Finally, one could argue that, consistent with expectancy theory (Porter and Lawler 1968; Vroom 1964), organizations and their key decision makers are motivated to act when they expect adequate rewards for doing so. In general, the greater the potential rewards, and the stronger the link between performance and rewards, the greater the motivation (Vroom 1964), unless the means for following the path are beyond the ability of the organization. Likewise, the stronger the perceived link between effort (e.g., implementing a specific hazard mitigation measure) and performance (e.g., increasing a hospital building's resistance to seismic forces), the greater the motivation to act. If an organization's decision makers do not believe that a given mitigation measure will increase significantly the organization's ability to achieve its goals (e.g., serve its community), then the mitigation measure is likely to be dismissed.

In the case of SB 1953, every hospital executive interviewed indicated that patient and staff life safety were essential goals. **No one believed that their hospital facilities posed a life safety threat.** Accordingly, any acceptable investment in hazard mitigation had to yield other important outcomes, such as reduced operating costs or increased revenue opportunities. Without these outcomes, how could a top executive justify expending millions of dollars on hazard mitigation that might be spent otherwise? Our interviews with hospital executives in Louisiana and Mississippi revealed a somewhat different understanding of extreme event consequences made salient by Hurricane Katrina. In nearly every case, hospital buildings in Louisiana and Mississippi remained standing and protected the life safety of their patients and staff in the wake of Katrina. What changed the perspective of these executives was not the immediate reaction of the hospital buildings and staff to Katrina, but the aftermath that included hospital evacuations and closures for months, even years. Some have yet to reopen, more than six years after the event. A closed hospital can neither tend its patients, nor cover its payroll or other expenses. The longer a hospital is closed, the harder and more expensive it is to reopen. As expressed by more than one Louisiana and Mississippi hospital executive, they now believe that hazard mitigation must go beyond the initial event, such that the hospital never closes. In brief, experience has taught these managers to see costs differently than they did before.

In order for an organization to act, to enact hazard mitigation measures, its decision makers must not only believe that the benefits of doing so will exceed the costs. They must also believe that the cost of present mitigation will be less than the cost of future recovery.

9.5 An Acceptable Solution Exists

Assuming that the three preceding prerequisites have been met, organizational decision makers must **perceive that there is an acceptable means to mitigate against extreme hazards, or nothing will be done**. A solution is not a solution unless decision makers know it exists and believe that it will be effective within their organizational context. There are at least three reasons why an organization might not be aware of workable solutions.

First, a workable solution may not yet exist. New problems, like broken steel welds in buildings, continue to surface, often as side effects of employing new technologies. It took quite a while, for example, to come up with the means to strengthen unreinforced masonry buildings that were cost-effective for owners.

Second, the inventory of workable (and affordable) solutions may be thin. Those old enough to have done business before xerographic copying machines will remember choosing between carbon paper and wet process copiers. Innovative ways to create multiple copies were developed, but at first, they were too expensive for all but the most affluent organizations. As costs dropped, more organizations were able to afford xerographic copiers. Now, many individuals have sophisticated copying machines in their homes for personal use. With respect to hazard mitigation, seismic isolation technology promises to protect both the structural and non-structural components of buildings, and yet the technology is perceived as too new and too expensive initially for many organizations in the United States to adopt. The exceptions include heritage buildings for which people are willing to spend more to minimize potential damage.

Third, even with continuing enhancements to communication systems such as the Internet, disseminating innovations takes time. Dissemination especially takes time when the innovation has been developed as proprietary property by an organization in the business of selling its mitigation techniques. Even when solutions are not secret, innovation dissemination and technology transfer can take a long time, as organizations may not routinely interact with relevant sources of hazard mitigation information (e.g., structural engineering firms). Returning to the case of seismic isolation technology, such technology is increasingly common in Japan, where seismically-isolated buildings fared well in the 1995 Great Hanshin (Kobe) earthquake. Such technology is not common in the United States, in part because it is not commonly taught in engineering curricula, but also because there are relatively few structural engineering firms that employ the technology and because there are fewer than 100 base-isolated buildings in the United States.

The ability to perceive an acceptable solution requires a belief that a problem is solvable. If an organization decides that a problem is intractable, the organization is likely to stop trying to understand the problem, and to cease efforts focused on finding a workable solution. Faced with the requirement to retrofit or rebuild their acute care hospital buildings at a cost of many millions of dollars, an organization bleeding red might well decide that there is simply no way to afford either a retrofit or a rebuild. The problem is unsolvable, and therefore unworthy of continued contemplation. Likewise, for the hospital organization that is physically limited in its remodeling or rebuilding opportunities, perhaps by the density of buildings adjacent to the hospital-owned property, the logistics of attempting a retrofit while staying in business may seem impossible to address. Again, the problem will be seen as unsolvable and unworthy of attention.

Intractability, of course, varies from time to time and place to place. Intractability often has less to do with complexity than it has to do with being locked into a perceptual paradigm that keeps one from seeing familiar things in new ways – ways that make obvious a solution to a situation that was otherwise impenetrable. So, what is intractable to some may not be intractable to others. Moreover, intractability can change to tractability with changes in the social, legal, or organizational environment. Some seismic safety advocates believe, for example, that if the insurance industry were to dramatically lower premiums for base-isolated buildings, then more building owners might see seismic isolation technology as affordable and ideal. Sometimes, intractability can change when new technologies become available. Again, research into seismic isolation technology continues with a view to reducing its cost and making it more applicable to existing buildings that must remain in use while being retrofitted. Sometimes, intractability can change when the problem is viewed by someone with a novel perspective. A new building owner who prefers to minimize a hospital's footprint and increase the number and capacity of clinics and surgery centers may decide that a hospital should relocate to another area, one less bound by adjacent properties and one that is less urban.

In any event, as long as an organization perceives a problem as intractable, little will likely be done toward implementing a solution. As one executive told us, "Given our location, our lack of resources, and our focused mission, there's no way for us to meet the hazard mitigation requirements of SB 1953." This executive believed the problem to be so intractable, that he no longer paid attention to what was happening with SB 1953. He asked more questions of us about the regulation than we asked of him in our interview.

9.6 The Organization Must Have the Capacity to Act

Even if all of the preceding four prerequisites are met, the organization may still not implement hazard mitigation measures. In the competition of issues and ideas for attention, mitigating natural hazard risks may not reach the top of the organizational agenda. It may be because other issues continue to crowd it out, because the organization lacks the capacity to do what it perceives necessary, or because the environment within which the organization would attempt implementation is itself dysfunctional.

9.6.1 The Organizational Agenda

"It's important, but we just have too much on our plate right now." How often is something like this said in the context of a formal organization faced with an array of important, urgent, and complex initiatives? Like individuals, organizations must set priorities and address issues based on criteria concerning what comes first. Often, unfortunately, operational concerns often consume time better spent on strategic assessment, so risks from extreme hazards perceived as having relatively low likelihood *this week* are pressed onto the back burner so today's "fire" may be put out.

As organizations expand their market share and increase in size, the number and variety of decisions competing for agenda space tends to increase, making it even more difficult for a big-ticket item like hazard mitigation to earn a spot on the top management team's agenda. Top managers must resolve myriad resource allocation issues in addition to setting and monitoring the organization's progress toward its strategic goals. Research on members of the top management team, also known as the organization's upper-echelons, has shown that the issues considered and the resolution of those issues depends in part on the functional background and experience of the top managers (Hambrick and Mason 1984). Getting an issue on the top management team's agenda is often a function of power differentials and advocacy (Arendt et al. 2005). Issues supported by powerful factions in the organization and championed by powerful advocates are more likely to be addressed (Finkelstein 1992). Unfortunately for those interested in hazard mitigation, members of the top management team are unlikely to have much experience in hazard mitigation. Instead, top managers tend to have functional expertise in finance, marketing, production (i.e., how the organization transforms inputs into outputs), human resources, R&D, and legal issues. Hazard mitigation does not fit neatly into any of these categories. As a result, the top management team is unlikely to have an "inner circle" hazard mitigation advocate. It's tough for an issue like hazard mitigation to get on an agenda when it's nobody's "baby."

9.6.2 Organizational Capacity: Financial Considerations

Any new activity requires an influx of additional resources or a reallocation of existing resources. In terms of extreme hazard mitigation, organizations must have (or must have access to) the financial means to invest in hazard mitigation. No additional or reallocated money means no hazard mitigation, no matter what. A common phrase heard in the healthcare industry is, "No margin, no mission." In other words, like all other organizations, hospitals need to generate revenue in order to perform their primary functions. Lack of revenue means lack of ability to attract inputs (e.g., staff members, equipment), which necessarily yields organizational entropy. To the extent that "no margin, no mission" accurately characterizes the hospital business (and we believe it does), we suggest that "no margin, no mitigation" accurately characterizes it as well. In considering the specific case of seismic mitigation, the remaining narrative on financial considerations is drawn from Alesch et al. (2005, pp. 44–48). We believe that it generalizes to any number of hazard mitigation types, and is not limited to the case of seismic mitigation. Whether an organization needs to retrofit against seismic hazard or hurricane and flooding hazard, resources must be found and allocated or reallocated. Rarely is mitigation against extreme hazards an inexpensive affair.

Perhaps the single greatest obstacle to implementing SB 1953 has been the unprecedented financial and structural upheaval in healthcare economics experienced since SB 1953 was passed. This upheaval made it financially impossible for most California hospitals to comply with the regulations in the years immediately following issuance of the rules, regardless of their ownership (e.g., investor owned, not-profit, or public).

When SB 1953 was enacted, many of California's healthcare organizations were generating profits or, in the case of not-for-profit and public hospitals, surpluses. By the late 1990s, however, more than 80% of California's healthcare organizations were losing money. More specifically, they were experiencing net operating losses (Shattuck Hammond 2001).

Two things happened to change the industry's financial situation and structure. First, the number of individuals participating in managed medical care increased dramatically during the second half of the 1990s, primarily as a response to rapidly escalating health insurance premiums. Between 1995 and 2005, a single decade, participation in managed care programs was projected to increase from 12.2 million Californians to 20.1 million (Shattuck Hammond 2001; Harrison and Montalvo 2002). For many decades, hospitals had charged patients for services received on a cost-plus basis. In the managed care environment, they were usually paid a fixed price for a service, regardless of their actual costs. Competition among HMOs for customers led them to cut payments to hospitals for treatment, often to less than the hospital's cost of providing the service.

Second, at the same time California HMOs were experiencing explosive growth, Medicare was experiencing problems associated with rising costs. The problem was not new, but it reached a point where something had to be done. Medical hospital costs per patient more than doubled from 1970 to 1975. They doubled again by 1980 (Shattuck Hammond 2001). The Federal government took action on the high cost of Medicare as part of the 1997 Federal Balanced Budget Act. It called for reducing Medicare expenditures by $215 billion over 5 years. Alas, the number of Medicare patients and the costs of treating them continued to increase. To meet the goal of cutting federal expenditures, Congress cut Medicare reimbursements to hospitals and healthcare professionals, often to levels below the cost of providing the services. To help achieve the balanced budget goal, hospitals were paid a fixed amount per discharge based on the patient's general diagnostic group, regardless of the actual cost of treating the patient.

All of this took place in an ongoing context of rapidly escalating costs for healthcare organizations. Dating to the early 1970s, the federal and state governments had been involved in trying to contain the rising costs of health care. Prior to 1986, for example, Congress had strongly encouraged states to enact "Certificate of Need" laws that required state health planning agencies to issue a permit before a health care facility could construct or expand, offer a new service, or purchase equipment exceeding a certain cost. The intent behind such "CON" laws was threefold: "to restrain escalating health care costs, prevent duplication of health resources, and yield equal access to quality health care at a reasonable cost." Such laws ultimately proved ineffectual in the fight to reduce health care costs. At the same time, both the cost of and the demand for contemporary diagnostic and treatment equipment were skyrocketing, particularly with the introduction of sophisticated new medications and advanced technologies. Moreover, the cost of supplies was increasing much faster than the Consumer Price Index.

Labor costs, which are a major component of hospital operating costs, were also increasing dramatically. Several forces drove the costs up. The number of Catholic nuns, devoted women who had provided nursing care for more than a century in hospitals with Catholic religious affiliations, declined precipitously. Since the nuns had worked for low pay, the rapid decline in their numbers had to be made up by hiring secular nurses at much higher cost. Simultaneously, California's population was swelling. More nurses were needed, but by the 1990s, both women and men had many professional occupational choices beyond nursing and teaching. Hospital work was demanding and did not pay competitively. The availability of licensed registered nurses declined in the face of increasing demand, even as pay increased.

Some hospitals, unable to staff themselves with the required number of nurses, found that they had to reduce the number of beds available for acute care. Administrators found themselves with declining revenues per patient, higher direct costs per patient, and the need to allocate large, fixed overhead costs across fewer patients.

The response by hospitals to this complex, dynamic, and troublesome combination of challenges was generally rational and rapid. Hospitals and physicians began to reorganize themselves to gain efficiencies. Hospitals sought to develop integrated delivery systems by aligning themselves with groups of physicians. This way, they thought, they could reduce costs and cope with "capitation," a form of payment to healthcare organizations from third-party payers that provides for a set amount of money per enrolled member per year, regardless of the number or types of treatment required.

At the same time, individual hospitals merged or affiliated with one another in hopes of realizing economies of scale (Spetz et al. 2000). Bigger, stronger corporations with more assets could presumably benefit from integrated management and operations. Hospital mergers swept the nation during the 1990s. They peaked from 1995 to1997, during which more than 680 hospital mergers were completed nationally.

Despite their efforts, California hospitals, on average, could not reduce costs quickly enough or deeply enough to make up for the reduction in revenue and the increases in the costs of equipment, labor, and materials. In 1999, California hospital median operating margins became negative. That is, by 1999, more than half of California's hospitals had negative cash flows. They were losing money.

In 1995, the median operating margin for California hospitals was 1.65% compared with 2.8% nationally. Operating margin, defined as "total operating revenue minus total operating expense," is considered "... a primary and 'early warning' indicator of the financial health of California's hospitals" (Shattuck Hammond 2001, p. 2). In part, operating margin is considered an important indicator because "operating margin directly and indirectly provides access to the capital required to sustain and/or grow a business in the future. Particularly in the capital-intensive hospital industry, access to capital (or lack thereof) determines future viability" (Shattuck Hammond 2001, p. 2). By 1999, California hospital median operating margins had become negative (–0.33%) while national median operating margins had declined, but remained positive (0.4%). In 1999, the top quartile of California's hospitals was outperforming the top 25% nationally, with operating margins of 5.7% compared to 5.0%, but the lowest quartile of California's hospitals was experiencing operating margins of –7.8% vs. –5.1% nationally (Shattuck Hammond 2001, p. 3).

The financial distress that developed in the second half of the 1990s was not shared equally by the all healthcare organizations. Hospitals most likely to have operating losses were small, owned by a local government (municipality, county, or special district), rural, not part of a healthcare system, and/or serving mostly poor patients. Those healthcare organizations most likely to still have positive operating margins were medium-large or large, investor-owned, urban, part of a system, and not receiving a disproportionately large proportion of poor patients as was the case with the public or Catholic hospitals (Shattuck Hammond 2001).

In the midst of the financial crisis facing more than half of California's healthcare organizations, the California legislature decided that requiring one nurse for every six patients in acute care units was not sufficient. In 2001, therefore, the legislature enacted a revised requirement for one nurse for every four patients in acute care facilities. It was, of course, unlikely that sufficient numbers of nurses existed in California to meet those new requirements. Consequently, healthcare organizations have been faced with further increasing pay for nurses to attract them from other states and from foreign countries. Alternatively, hospital organizations could reduce their available beds to meet the standards. Whatever the medical merits of the new nursing ratio requirement, the financial burden for a very significant number of hospitals could be expected to further depress net operating revenues.

In this milieu, healthcare organizations with many facilities had more flexibility and options. Such organizations could presumably afford short-term losses in one or a few facilities, as long as other facilities generated sufficient revenues to cover any losses incurred by the organization overall. Likewise, healthcare organizations that were investor-owned typically had more flexibility and options than did not-for-profit and publicly owned hospitals. Some readers will leap to the assumption that investor-owned hospitals are more efficient than not-for-profit or public hospitals. That is not necessarily the case. What is more likely is that investor-owned healthcare organizations can generally choose where, how, and to whom to provide service. They are in a better position to locate in upscale markets and are able to focus on providing services that have favorable reimbursements from insurance and Medicare payers. Further, they are in a better position to lure and retain medical specialists whose expertise is associated with higher revenues (e.g., orthopedics, plastic surgery).

Public hospitals and many not-for-profit hospitals rarely have the option to "cherry pick" their markets and customers. Indeed, they are often serving the customers who are least able to pay. Not-for-profit hospitals typically have missions to serve particular neighborhoods or communities, whether they are secular or religiously based. As such, while not-for-profit and public hospitals might benefit by adopting more of the efficiency-oriented practices associated with investor-owned hospitals, they could not implement all of them and still be true to their missions. Moreover, neither the not-for-profits nor the public hospitals could segment the market as aggressively as the investor-owned hospitals could. Finally, in considering especially the case of the not-for-profit and the public hospitals, local governments have suffered with their own fiscal problems and have been limited in their ability to provide sufficient funds for either contemporary capital infrastructure or preventive maintenance.

These financial and structural changes in the healthcare industry have a great deal to do with the initial responses of healthcare organizations to SB 1953. Hospitals experiencing financial hemorrhaging or barely surviving were not likely able to justify spending money on seismic retrofitting, at least in the short run. At the same time, healthcare organizations able to remain profitable may have been in a position to benefit from the mandated seismic improvements. The costs of retrofits provide legitimate reasons to eliminate "loser" hospital facilities and complexes, by either selling or closing them. Since so many healthcare organizations were in difficult financial straits, this also presented profitable healthcare organizations with the opportunity to strengthen their market positions by acquiring desirable facilities and market locations from financially strapped organizations. One might expect, in this environment, that the largest and most profitable organizations might greatly expand their market share. Unfortunately, one could also expect those organizations to expand their market share by building on the profitable areas of healthcare, leaving those procedures and services with low or below cost reimbursements to public and not-for-profit hospitals.

The upshot of all this was that, depending on their fiscal position and their primary organizational objectives, it made sense for some healthcare organizations to support SB 1953 and to move forward with compliance on schedule. Compliance would be easier for them because they would have had a variety of options for dealing with inadequate buildings, and because they could benefit organizationally from the difficulties stressing other healthcare organizations. It was to their clear advantage to address their buildings' seismic issues, and then declare to potential customers and coveted medical providers that they were "ahead of the curve" – both in terms of seismic issues, and in terms of updated facilities overall. Other organizations might have been barely able to comply. Still others may have been unable to at all.

Could healthcare organizations have borrowed or otherwise generated sufficient funds to finance the mandated retrofits or replacement? It appears that they could not. Standard and Poors noted that "cash flow generation for a high percentage of California hospitals is insufficient to finance any significant increase in capital expenditures" (Harrison et al. 2001, cited in Shattuck Hammond). Shattuck Hammond analysts compared credit ratio data for the sum of California hospitals and for the overall median with Moody's national median ratios. The ratios compared with Baa credits, the lowest investment grade bond rating offered by Moody's. The lower the bond rating, the higher the interest that must be paid to sell the bonds.

Importantly, the State of California has an office to help healthcare organizations borrow money. It works to find the best rates, using the State's bond rating, but few hospitals sought help from the agency to borrow money for retrofits, in large part because their precarious financial positions made it difficult for them to demonstrate credit-worthiness. Given the negative cash flow situation that more than half of California's hospitals were experiencing during the late 1990s, it appears as though they would have considerable difficulty servicing the debt, even if they could float a bond issue. Paradoxically, those investor-owned and not-for-profit healthcare facilities with strong cash positions and positive cash flows typically would not need the State's services to obtain favorable bond rates or to meet the costs of meeting SB 1953.

9.6.3 *The Organizational Environment*

The environment within which an organization attempts to reduce its hazard risk is critically important to successful implementation. Organizational environments can range from placid and predictable to convoluted and chaotic (Emery and Trist 1965). Environmental factors that may affect an organization include the industry, suppliers, consumers, socio-cultural aspects, technology, political-legal aspects, human resources, and physical resources. The greater the number of and the more interconnected the environmental factors expected to directly affect an organization, the more complex its task environment. This complexity, along with the rate of change in these factors (dynamism), and the lack or abundance of needed resources (munificence), determine the relative amount of environmental uncertainty faced by the organization (Dess and Beard 1984).

When organizational environments are highly unpredictable and extremely complex, the chances of successful policy implementation may diminish appreciably. Scholars of implementation concluded this long ago. In 1973, Pressman and Wildavsky concluded that "the multiplicity of participants and perspectives combined to produce a formidable obstacle course ... When a program depends on so many actors, there are numerous possibilities for disagreement and delay ... (G)iven a large number of clearance points manned by diverse and independent participants, the probability of a program achieving its goals is low" (pp. 102–110). We agree. The probability of successful, timely implementation of extreme hazard mitigation is inversely related to the complexity of the implementation process, the number of actors participating in the process, the number of sign-offs required, and the diversity of interests and priorities among the actors.

References

Alesch DJ, Petak WJ (1986) The politics and economics of earthquake hazard mitigation. University of Colorado, Boulder

Alesch DJ, Arendt LA, Petak WJ (2005) Seismic safety in California hospitals: assessing an attempt to accelerate the replacement or seismic retrofit of older hospital facilities. Multidisciplinary Center for Earthquake Engineering Research, University of Buffalo, State University of New York. Technical report MCEER-05-0006, 6 June 2005

Arendt LA, Priem RL, Ndofor HA (2005) A CEO-Adviser model of strategic decision making. J Manage 31(5):680–699

Boone C, Van Olffen W, Van Witteloostuijn A (2005) Team locus-of-control composition, leadership structure, information acquisition, and financial performance: a business simulation study. Acad Manage J 48:889–909

Dess GG, Beard DW (1984) Dimensions of organizational task environments. Adm Sci Q 29:52–73

Emery FE, Trist EL (1965) The causal texture of organizational environments. Hum Relat 18:21–32

Finkelstein S (1992) Power in top management teams: dimensions, measurement, and validation. Acad Manage J 35:505–538

Hambrick D, Mason P (1984) Upper echelons: the organization as a reflection of its top managers. Acad Manage Rev 9:193–206
Harrison MA, Montalvo C (2002) The financial health of California hospitals: a looming crisis. Health Aff 21(1):15–23
Harrison MG, Montalvo CC, Fiorella SL (2001) The financial health of California hospitals. Shattuck Hammons Partners
March JG, Simon HA (1958) Organizations. Wiley, New York
March JG, Olsen JP (1973) Ambiguity and choice in organizations. Universitetsforlaget, Bergen
Petak WJ, Alesch DJ (2004) Organizational decision making with respect to extreme events: healthcare organizations respond to California's SB 1953. In research progress and accomplishments: 2003–2004 (MCEER-04-SP01). University of Buffalo, State University of New York, Multidisciplinary Center for Earthquake Engineering Research, Buffalo, May 2004
Porter LW, Lawler EE (1968) Managerial attitudes and performance. Dorsey Press, Homewood
Pressman J, Wildavsky A (1973) Implementation: how great expectations in Washington are dashed in Oakland. University of California Press, Berkeley
Rotter JB (1966) Generalized expectancies for internal versus external control of reinforcement. Psychological monographs, Complete number 609
Shattuck Hammond Partners (2001) The financial health of California hospitals, July
Shea GP, Guzzo RA (1987) Group effectiveness: what really matters? Sloan Manage Rev 28(3):25–31
Spetz J, Mitchell S, Seago J (2000) The growth of multihospital firms in California. Health Aff 19(4):24–30
Vroom V (1964) Work and motivation. Wiley, New York
Woo G (2002) Natural catastrophe probable maximum loss. British Actuarial Journal, vol. 8, Part V

Chapter 10
Organizational Differences in Hazard Mitigation Investment Decision Making: Inside the Organization

In this chapter, we present three critical categories of factors that we believe influence whether, why, and how individual hospital organizations make extreme hazard mitigation investment decisions. Each category reflects internal organizational concerns and perspectives.

We describe each category from a theoretical perspective, drawing on relevant academic literature. Then, we augment our description of each category with examples drawn from our qualitative research. As stated earlier, the examples capture decision making by California hospitals facing the decision to comply with SB 1953, by hospitals facing seismic threats in Oregon and Washington, and by hospitals facing hurricane threats in Louisiana and Mississippi. In this way, our examples illustrate the impact of the critical categories beyond the environment of SB 1953.

The three categories are intended to be illustrative, rather than exhaustive. The unit of analysis is the individual organization and its key decision makers, usually the members of the top management team (i.e., the CEO, CFO, COO, and other members of the C-suite).

10.1 Organizational Leadership Predictors

Management scholars (e.g., Hambrick and Mason 1984; Wiersema and Bantel 1992) have argued that the characteristics of those occupying an organization's upper-echelons condition the organization's decision-making process and outcomes. For our purposes, an organization's upper-echelons include the top manager (e.g., CEO) and those managers who report directly to the top manager (e.g., the COO, CFO, CIO). Other than an organization's Board of Directors, the individuals who comprise an organization's upper-echelons, or top management team, are expected to exert the greatest amount of influence with respect to strategic decisions, including all major capital expenditure decisions.

D.J. Alesch et al., *Natural Hazard Mitigation Policy: Implementation, Organizational Choice, and Contextual Dynamics*, Environmental Hazards,
DOI 10.1007/978-94-007-2235-4_10,

We view two individual characteristics as particularly relevant to the consideration of hazard mitigation investment decisions: functional backgrounds and previous disaster experiences. First, we expect that top managers' **functional backgrounds** likely affect the way they perceive the hazard mitigation problem and potential solutions. Functional background is understood to include the knowledge and expertise that one acquires because of experience in a particular functional domain (e.g., finance, operations). Such knowledge and expertise accrue to individuals through both their formal education and their actual work experience. While some individuals' functional backgrounds may include several disciplines, we expect that most individuals' functional backgrounds consist of one or two complementary disciplines (e.g., finance and accounting).

Previous research suggests that functional background affects managerial perceptions, at least with respect to perceptions of organizational effectiveness (e.g., Waller et al. 1995). Thus, top managers with a functional background in finance might be expected to view potential decision opportunities through an economic lens, and to rely primarily on economic criteria, such as return on investment, when choosing among potential action alternatives. In the case of hospitals, top managers with a functional background in patient care might be expected to view potential decision opportunities through a relational lens, and to rely primarily on relational criteria, such as patient satisfaction, when choosing among potential action alternatives.

Similarly, previous research suggests that functional background affects resource allocation decisions (Barker and Mueller 2002). Top managers with a functional background in marketing might be expected to allocate more resources for organizational R&D. In the case of hospitals, top managers with a functional background in finance might be expected to allocate more resources to projects associated with positive cash flow.

In fact, the number of hospital executives having functional backgrounds in business, especially finance, appears to have increased over the past two decades (Molpus 2004). An increasing percentage of hospital CEOs have an MBA or its equivalent in addition to or in lieu of an MD. As such, we expect that strategic decisions made in hospitals are at least as likely to be made in light of economic criteria, specifically return on investment, as they are to be made in light of relational criteria, such as patient satisfaction. Specifically, in organizations having a high proportion of top management team members with a functional background in accounting or finance, top managers are likely to emphasize **economic criteria** (e.g., ROI) when they make hazard mitigation investment decisions.

In fact, our interviews revealed that a significant number of C-level decision makers had backgrounds in business (finance) and health administration. Relatively few C-level administrators had risen to top-level management as patient care staff members (i.e., physicians, nurses). Instead, most were career administrators who had been promoted within their own hospitals or across hospitals following predictable career paths. For example, most of the CEOs we interviewed had served previously as COOs or CFOs. All had advanced degrees in administration of some form. Consequently, all discussed the importance of **financial ratios** when making capital decisions, and all discussed the need for hazard mitigation investments to have a meaningful impact on the "bottom line." At the same time, all were quick to note that their interests were with patient care and safety as much as with the bottom line.

The following case illustrates the impact of top managers' functional background on their hazard mitigation investment decision making. The hospital is part of a larger corporation that owns hospitals in several states. The corporation is in the business of making money by providing health care services. The corporation chose this particular location to purchase a hospital because of the market there: It has a growing population, other acute care hospital facilities are not adequate to serve the area, and the area is above average in income with an above average rate of insured customers. The decision was made to acquire facilities in this location even though profit margins for hospitals in California are lower than elsewhere, partly because reimbursements are comparatively low and the costs of operation, including nursing staff, are particularly high.

The corporation makes the critical, strategic decisions, including the location of new hospital facilities, acquisitions, and facility sales, but the administrators of local facilities are important participants in capital decisions. The individual hospitals in the corporation develop operating and capital budgets that are submitted to the corporate level. There is extensive interaction between the corporate offices and individual hospitals. Large capital investment decisions are made at the corporate level; the corporation then provides funds for the improvements. Criteria for investment in individual facilities include meeting the needs for patient safety, meeting regulations, and generating revenue, in that order. Other criteria are secondary. Individual hospitals are charged with complying with their annual budgets. Budget status is tracked monthly and variances must be explained and addressed.

The management staff is professional and may move within the corporation or among individual facilities. At this facility, most members of the senior management team have graduate degrees in their area of specialization (e.g., finance, development, nursing). The dominant area of functional expertise is financial and strategic management. To some extent, this hospital's top managers are "hired guns" who have established themselves as knowing how to maximize the revenue generated by a given hospital location while also minimizing costs. Their job is to provide corporate management with a local connection and operational oversight. The corporation's top managers are interested in financial results. Hospitals that deliver financial results are retained with the corporate family; hospitals that do not deliver financial results are sold or, in a worst-case scenario, closed. The criteria that drive "buy-sell" decisions are financial. This is not to say that the hospitals' top managers are not concerned with patient care and well-being. To the contrary, patient care is seen as critical to the production of financial results. Simply put, the corporation and its top managers are concerned with patient care and financial results; if the latter aren't being produced or if they don't seem likely to be produced in the relatively near future, then the hospital will no longer be part of the corporation.

The single-building hospital facility acquired by this corporation does not meet the SB 1953 structural standards and the corporation has no plans to upgrade the facility. According to the current facility's top managers, "(The current facility) is being replaced by a new facility. That was our plan all along." The existing facility is inadequate in terms of size, operating characteristics, and infrastructure, so the hospital administration has advised the corporate office to avoid making any capital improvements to it. It also suffered from deferred maintenance by the previous owner. Plans are well underway to create a new facility in a nearby location. "The SB 1953 regulations have nothing to do with it. We need a better facility than the one occupied by the hospital we bought, a facility that will allow us to differentiate ourselves and provide higher-end services." While the current facility is not considered financially viable, the area is growing, and demand for hospital services are expected to increase as well. The area's new population is not poor, and positive financial results are expected once the new facility is built and operational. Capital for the new hospital will be made available through the national corporation.

In addition to top managers' functional background, we expect that top managers' previous experience with disasters likely affects the way they perceive the hazard mitigation problem and potential solutions. The first of Petak and Alesch's (2004, p. 127) prerequisites to organizational action is that the organization (i.e., the organization's top managers) "must be *aware* of a threat, opportunity, or challenge from its relevant environment and *believe* it to be salient to the organization" (*emphasis added*). Experience is widely regarded as a fundamental source of knowledge and subsequent action. Whether top managers believe that a particular hazard is likely to befall their organization is expected to depend in part on whether those managers have previous experience with the particular hazard (Hess and Arendt 2006), and on whether those managers believe that the circumstances of their current hospital (e.g., building type, location near a known earthquake fault) align with the circumstances of the hospitals or other organizations to which they belonged during a previous disaster. In brief, organizations are more likely to make hazard mitigation investments if their top managers have **experience with disasters** and if the top managers' assessment of their acute care hospital facility suggests that it is at risk of being damaged in the event of an extreme hazard.

The impact of disaster experience varies depending on *when* the experience occurred and how *traumatic* the experience was. Research suggests that the recency of an event affects its potential to influence judgment and decision making (Hertwig et al. 2004). Accordingly, the more recent one's disaster experience, then the more salient the threat, and the more concerned one is likely to be about future disasters. As time goes by, the disaster's saliency fades, and it may have significantly less effect on current decision making. As time goes by, the disaster is perceived as an aberration rather than as something to be anticipated and managed. Research also suggests that the traumatic nature of an event influences its future impact on behavior and decision making. The more traumatic the disaster experience, then the more salient the threat, and the more concerned one is likely to be about future disasters. Hence, organizations are more likely to make hazard mitigation investments if their top managers have **recent** experience with disasters and/or if their experience with disasters has been **traumatic**.

When asked about their experience with disasters, the hospital administrators from California all seemed knowledgeable with respect to seismic safety in California.

Many had lived in California for many years, and had experienced their fair share of earthquakes, as had many of the administrators at hospitals in Oregon and Washington. We were surprised to discover that while many of these administrators were concerned about seismic safety and hazard mitigation, others conveyed a surprising lack of urgency.

In thinking about the perceptions of this latter group, we conclude that their actual experiences with disasters in general, and earthquakes in particular, may be a major contributor to their general non-interest in making hazard mitigation investments. Though it may seem counterintuitive at first, this non-interest makes sense when one understands that: (1) none of these executives' earthquake experiences had been associated with patient deaths or even injuries resulting from a failed hospital building, and (2) many of these hospital executives perceived their hospital buildings to be secure from major structural damage from earthquakes. More than one hospital executive pointed at us and asked, "Do you know how many patients have died in a California hospital due to an earthquake in the last 30 years? None!"

In brief, while many of these administrators believe in earthquakes, they don't think that any future earthquakes will cause major problems for their facilities or for their staff or patients. They don't think that any future earthquake will be as bad as seismologists and seismic engineers seem to think. Their perception is undoubtedly influenced, at least in part, by the relatively long period of time since the last U.S. earthquake to cause significant damage. That earthquake, the Northridge earthquake, occurred in 1994, 10–14 years before our interviews were conducted. Their perception is also a function of whether they were in charge of any hospitals in the Los Angeles area when the Northridge earthquake occurred. Relatively few of the Los Angeles-area hospital administrators we interviewed were also administrators in the area when the Northridge earthquake struck more than a decade earlier.

Interviews with Louisiana and Mississippi hospital administrators in early 2007 and in 2008 revealed a different level of urgency with respect to hazard mitigation planning and investment. These interviews occurred about 18 months after Hurricane Katrina ravaged the Mississippi Coast and several parishes in Louisiana, including most notably Orleans Parish. Interviewees were administrators who had been with their hospitals before, during, and after Katrina.

The hospital administrators in Louisiana and Mississippi who led their hospitals through Hurricane Katrina and its aftermath were actively interested in enhancing their organization's resilience to future extreme hazards, specifically hurricanes and floods. They had witnessed firsthand the lethal effects of a major natural disaster on their facilities and on their ability to serve their community and provide patient care, and they were committed to avoiding a similar fate in the future. Administrators whose hospitals had been evacuated and closed described their fervent desire to "never close" their hospitals again; those whose hospitals remained open described their fervent desire to avoid the need to close. Closing a hospital is costly; reopening a hospital – cleaning, restaffing, restocking – is incredibly costly. The New Orleans experience illustrates how costly such a reopening can be. More than six years later, some hospitals are still shuttered, and will probably never reopen.

This latter point relates to the degree of trauma associated with disasters, and the impact of that trauma on future hazard mitigation investments. In both Louisiana and along the Mississippi Coast, the devastation wrought by Katrina was complete. Public infrastructure was irreparably damaged, schools were closed and destroyed, residences were ruined and later gutted or demolished, and businesses were shuttered. As described by Alesch and colleagues (Alesch et al. 2001), the residents experienced a "360° disaster." Everywhere they looked, they saw destruction. Every newspaper and every television news show talked about the lingering effects of Katrina.

With flood lines and slabs without houses everywhere serving as a daily reminder, it was no surprise that hospital administrators were keenly aware of the need to make hazard mitigation investments. Also serving as a reminder were the numerous requests for administrators to describe for various audiences their Katrina experience, how they addressed the disaster, and how they were planning to mitigate potential hazards in the future. Several major hurricanes (e.g., Rita, Gustav) after Katrina reinforced the need to plan and spend money on hazard mitigation.

When asked what they thought would be the best catalyst for hazard mitigation investment decision making, everyone we interviewed, regardless of their location, said "a major earthquake" or "a major hurricane." The statement was neither flippant nor sarcastic. These individuals simply reaffirmed that many people respond most vigorously to experienced threats, especially those with traumatic and lasting consequences. Nothing creates urgency and a desire to act like a real disaster.

There is no question that Katrina made salient the need for Louisiana and Mississippi hospital administrators to engage in disaster planning and hazard mitigation investment decision making. Interestingly, they remained focused on allocating resources to mitigate against the one extreme event that had impacted negatively their facility, significantly more so than they focused on allocating resources to mitigate against hazards not yet experienced by their hospital or by similar hospitals. Hence, 18 months after Hurricane Katrina, many of these hospitals had not yet turned their avid attention to issues such as pandemic flu. They were still concerned with mitigating against the "next" Hurricane Katrina, an extreme event that they now viewed as likely and "real." As more than one administrator told us, they hadn't yet addressed all of the needs associated with hurricane mitigation, and couldn't allocate resources to mitigating other potential disasters.

10.2 Organizational Strategy Predictors

The particular business-level strategy adopted by an organization consequently affects or should affect decisions around resource allocation (Porter 1980). Each of Porter's (1980) generic strategies – differentiation, cost leadership, and focus – makes different assumptions about the market to be served, and the approach to serving the chosen market. An organization adopting a differentiation strategy seeks to distinguish itself in the industry and secure profits by means of producing or delivering a unique, premium product or service to a broad-based market. As described by the head of one for-profit hospital organization in California, "We compete for quality physicians and we have a reputation for quality patient care. We must be at the "head of the pack" if we want to survive financially and to continue to serve our clientele." If successful, the organization pursuing a differentiation strategy should be able to charge a premium price for its product or service. An organization adopting a cost leadership strategy seeks to achieve market dominance through relentless cost cutting and subsequent production or delivery of the lowest-price products or services, also to a broad-based market. An organization adopting a focus strategy chooses either a differentiation or a cost-leadership strategy and applies it to a niche market.

Whether and to what extent an organization decides to invest in hazard mitigation would seem to depend in part on whether the organization's decision makers believed that the investment would align with the organization's chosen strategy. In the case of hospitals, for example, those with a **differentiation strategy** might be expected to invest in hazard mitigation only if such mitigation would help the organization position itself as offering something "special" to end-users. Offering something "special" is prerequisite to charging a premium for one's products or services. Since hazard mitigation, especially seismic hazard mitigation, tends to be invisible to the typical hospital user, we would expect to see it occur in the context of visible changes. As suggested earlier, we would expect to see hazard mitigation linked to capital projects that provide end-users (e.g., doctors, patients) with tangible premium benefits, such as newly constructed "boutique-style" bed towers boasting all private rooms.

Hospitals with a **cost-leadership strategy** might be expected to invest in hazard mitigation only if such mitigation would help the organization position itself as "spending money now to save money later." Considering expenses in terms of their ability to reduce costs is prerequisite to being a low-cost leader. Since hazard mitigation, especially seismic mitigation, tends to be expensive in terms of capital and ongoing operating expenses, we would expect to see it occur in the context of enhancing efficiency. For example, we would expect to see hazard mitigation linked to capital projects that enhance hospital efficiency, such as newly constructed or remodeled bed towers that are LEED certified.

In general, then, we expect that hospital executives would be most likely to invest in hazard mitigation that serves a broader purpose, that of helping the organization pursue its overall strategy. Similarly, we expect that hospital executives would be most likely to invest in hazard mitigation that aligns with a pre-existing facilities plan or strategy. If a hospital was planning already to rebuild its bed towers, for example, it seems likely that investing in hazard mitigation at the same time would be relatively straightforward. More than one hospital executive with whom we spoke described SB 1953 as something that "just happened" to align with plans the hospital already had for its physical plant. "We were planning to build a new acute care bed tower anyway." Likewise, if a hospital were planning already to alter its facilities to conform to ADA or other regulations, again, it seems likely that investing in hazard mitigation at the same time would be relatively straightforward. In general, then, to the extent that hazard mitigation investments support or "piggyback" the organization's overall business strategy or facility plans, we expect greater acceptance of and willingness to make hazard mitigation investments. Overall, we believe that organizations are more likely to make hazard mitigation investments if the association between hazard mitigation and the organization's strategy (i.e., differentiation, cost leadership, focus) or existing facility plans is high.

Throughout our interviews, and often without necessarily realizing it, hospital executives discussed their business-level strategies, and the relationship of those strategies to hazard mitigation investments. The hospitals most likely to have plans drawn up for rebuilding or retrofitting their acute care hospital buildings were those that had started thinking about doing so in advance of SB 1953. In other words, the need to invest in hazard mitigation in response to SB 1953 just happened to coincide with existing plans to alter a hospital's physical plant. Or, SB 1953 was the catalyst that helped a community commit to providing the financial support needed to execute an existing rebuilding plan.

Hospitals pursuing differentiation strategies tended to be already interested in either modifying their existing physical facilities or in building modern facilities. SB 1953 had no measurable impact on their capital investment decision, since these hospital organizations planned to alter their facilities before the statutory catalyst of SB 1953 was introduced. Hospital managers recognize that building new hospital facilities can take considerable time from conception and design to opening, often more than a decade. Hospital organizations that were already planning to upgrade their facilities had a competitive advantage over those that decided to upgrade in response to SB 1953.

Despite some perceptions to the contrary, the hospital industry is fiercely competitive. Hospitals compete for patients. They compete for doctors. They compete for nurses. They compete for other staff members. They compete for insurance partnerships. They compete for physical and material resources. They compete with each other, and they compete with other organizations offering similar services, for example, surgery centers. In order to compete effectively, they must possess some core competence, something that sets them apart from their competitors. Even hospital organizations in rural areas, hospitals that do not have other hospitals in their immediate geographic area, compete. Again, they compete for doctors. They compete for nurses. They compete for other staff members. And so it goes. All hospitals compete. Even the public and non-profit hospitals compete, because the resources they need to ensure their survival are desired by other hospital and related organizations.

The idea that hospitals compete was supported in interview after interview. If it weren't for competition, hospitals would not have to buy commercials, billboards, and other visible marketing media to secure resources. They would not be interested in establishing a social media presence. They would not have to ask staff members to sign non-compete clauses. They would not offer duplicative services within given geographical areas, services that are expensive and that draw down each hospital organization's profit or surplus.

Accordingly, hospitals must offer modern patient rooms, both private and large. Hospitals must offer modern surgical facilities, complete with complex video and computer-guided equipment. Electronic monitoring and record-keeping devices must interface seamlessly with other non-structural elements (e.g., HVAC). The walls and ceilings must be able to accommodate the requisite piping, wiring, cable, etc.

If hospitals pursuing differentiation strategies were considering facility upgrades before SB 1953 went into effect, what about the hospitals pursuing cost-leadership strategies? Were they also interested in facility upgrades? The answer is "yes" and "no." Like their differentiating competitors, hospitals pursuing a cost-leadership strategy are expected to offer modern facilities in order to be competitive. Unlike their differentiating competitors, hospitals pursuing a cost-leadership strategy weigh the appropriateness of resource allocations in the context of their ability to reduce costs. After all, the cost leader competes by offering services of equivalent value for less. The more money saved on facilities, for example, the more money available to recruit (and pay for) essential resources, such as doctors practicing higher-margin specialties (e.g., orthopedics).

Most of the cost-leaders interviewed did not have sufficient resources available to undertake a substantial facility upgrade or to replace their facilities. Hence, while they were able to appreciate the potential for reduced operating costs afforded by a new or upgraded facility, they did not have access to the resources needed to build such a facility.

More than one hospital executive, both differentiators and cost-leaders, wanted to know why hazard mitigation was not being treated like other regulations that affected buildings. For example, everyone understood that major changes to existing facilities would be accompanied by the need to alter those facilities in line with ADA and similar building regulations. Rather than require hospitals to rebuild or retrofit facilities outside the normal replacement cycle, when the cost of doing so would be excessive (e.g., since the building may not have been fully depreciated), why not require hospitals to incorporate seismic hazard mitigation into any major changes? That way, the decision to upgrade or replace a building would be integrated with the rest of the hospital's strategic and capital decision-making process, and would therefore be driven by the hospital's strategic priorities (e.g., differentiation vs. cost-leadership). After all, these executives reasoned, shouldn't strategic priorities drive capital decision making, rather than building regulations?

One case illustrates the preceding narrative especially well.

The hospital in this case is a stand-alone. It is an old hospital, located in an old, higher income suburb. The hospital is governed by a board of directors, which is self-perpetuating; i.e., the board itself names replacement board members as seats become vacant. The board, drawn primarily from the community, plays a key role in the organization. It meets monthly, engages in discussions with staff about both policy and operating issues, and works successfully to find philanthropic support for the hospital.

The staff is highly professional. The top management team has graduate training in finance and healthcare administration and extensive relevant experience. The tenure of corporate level executives varies considerably, but all have held high-level positions for some time.

The hospital's business-level strategy is to differentiate itself from other healthcare organizations. It has developed a reputation as a prestigious community hospital and strives to maintain that reputation. It works hard to identify itself with the community. The hospital has a strong balance sheet and bond rating. It was able to withstand the financial turmoil of the 1990s and to begin generating an operating surplus a few years ago. The operating surplus is small and will not support major capital investments or service a substantial debt load by itself.

The buildings that comprise this hospital campus were built over many decades. Many of them have been upgraded over the years, but the older, primary acute care building is not compliant with SB 1953s structural standards. Years before SB 1953 was enacted, the hospital initiated a planning and development program that would, coincidentally, make the acute care facility compliant. SB 1953 has not driven the replacement of the acute care facility; replacement is being driven by the desire for a larger, more efficient, and more "user-friendly" facility – one that will allow the hospital to continue to differentiate itself from other hospitals in terms of services offered and quality. The hospital sees the SB 1953 mandate as accelerating some construction, but complying with SB 1953 "is an afterthought." The principal problem with the hospital's construction program is financial. The operating margin alone will not support the investment. Consequently, the hospital has been seeking philanthropic gifts as a mainstay of the capital investment program. No matter what, the organization is committed to building a new facility, one that will meet the current seismic codes and allow the organization to differentiate itself from its competition.

10.3 Economic Predictors

As described by Sharfman and his colleagues (2000, p. 280), organizations cannot "operate in the long term at a price point lower or a cost point higher than the intersection of marginal costs and marginal revenues - P." This assertion will remain accurate whether the organization is investor or equity-owned, not-for-profit, or public. Organizations must cover their costs. Without an adequate revenue stream, organizations cannot acquire sufficient resources or inputs to sustain their core transformation processes. Doctors, nurses, and other staff members cannot be hired and paid competitive wages. Medical equipment cannot be purchased and maintained. Likewise, furniture and office equipment cannot be purchased and maintained. Mechanical, electrical, and plumbing equipment cannot be installed. Without adequate inputs or well functioning transformation processes, organizations cannot produce or deliver quality outputs. Patients will not get the care they need, buildings and equipment will fall into disrepair, and staff turnover will be high. Failure to deliver quality outputs over a sustained period will cause the organization to enter a state of entropy, or organizational death (Katz and Kahn 1978).

In order to change this price or cost point, organizations must change something about their core production process such that their marginal production or transaction costs are lowered, or they are able to charge prices above "P." Accomplishing such a change is done through alterations to design, introduction of new or more efficient technology, or creative efforts of people (Evans 1997). Organizations must either simplify or make lean their production or service operation in order to reduce their costs, or they must augment their product or service such that consumers are willing to pay a premium for something they believe is unique. These operational activities are closely aligned with the business-level strategies of cost-leadership and differentiation. They can also align with corporate-level strategies such as vertical integration, which seeks to reduce transaction costs, and related or unrelated diversification, which can enable deeper or broader market penetration.

Unless hazard mitigation investments allow the organization to lower its costs or raise its prices, the organization is unlikely to make such investments. Importantly, hazard mitigation investments represent only one of a large array of potential expenditures that might yield lowered costs or increased prices. In the specific case of acute care hospitals, the possibilities for capital expenditures are many, and most represent additions to the acute care setting that are far more visible than hazard mitigation to both internal users (e.g., physicians, nurses, administrators) and external users (e.g., patients, patient family members). Illustratively, physicians are more likely to see the value in procuring a new MRI machine that can be used to facilitate caring for more people better than they are likely to see the value in retrofitting a building with base isolation to enhance structural resistance to seismic forces.

Likewise, potential patients are more likely to be impressed with private rooms and space for family members to sleep than by seemingly invisible strengthening of a hospital's lateral resistance to seismic forces. In the end, the opportunity to invest in hazard mitigation will compete with several other investment possibilities, most likely unfavorably, since hazard mitigation investments, both structural and non-structural, are generally not visible to most hospital users. Accordingly, organizations may want to link hazard mitigation activities to more visible enhancements (e.g., remodeled bed towers that boast larger private rooms, building a "green" building) that either lower the cost or enable price increases. In general, we suggest that organizations are more likely to make hazard mitigation investments if the hazard mitigation investments (or the investments to which they are linked) **decrease operating or transaction costs** or allow the organization to **increase its prices**.

The regulatory and socio-economic environment can be expected to affect the extent to which an organization's key decision makers consider economics in their hazard mitigation investment decision-making process. For example, regulations with a focus other than hazard mitigation that potentially affect an organization's operating or transaction costs are likely to divert attention and resources away from hazard mitigation investments. In the case of hospitals in California, regulations around increasingly smaller staffing ratios for nurses have directed attention toward the costs associated with compensation and benefits, a major component of a hospital's operating budget, and away from the costs associated with hazard mitigation. The negative impact of such regulation on hazard mitigation investment decision making is made all the more potent by three factors: the regulation's immediacy – the staffing ratios must be achieved in short order; by its visibility – both internal and external users can ascertain for themselves whether the regulation seems to be met; and by its support from a large group of vocal advocates (e.g., nurses) embedded in the affected communities.

Likewise, the socio-economic environment facing some hospitals greatly limits their ability to address high-cost capital investments such as seismic retrofits or new building. The socio-economic reality for many hospitals, especially urban and rural hospitals, is that many of their patients will be chronically and seriously ill, under-insured or uninsured, and unable to pay. These hospitals struggle to cover their basic operating costs while fulfilling their critical mission of serving the very poor. For these hospitals to consider major capital investments of any kind is a "pipe dream." An example of a large hospital serving an urban and largely poor population was Charity Hospital in New Orleans, Louisiana. Located in the city's Central Business District, "Big Charity" was the Level I trauma center for the New Orleans metropolitan area. Its primary mission was to care for the city's poorest citizens. Few were able to pay for the care received. Shuttered after Hurricane Katrina, the 1939-built hospital was ill-suited to delivering modern medicine before Katrina, and unsuitable for providing care after being severely flooded and left without power and air conditioning for more than a month.

Although the hospital's administrators had discussed their desire to build a new Charity Hospital before Katrina, there was no funding for such a massive undertaking. Like many other urban and very rural hospitals, there simply wasn't enough money available for capital investments because the relatively small amount of money that did flow into the hospital for patient care was applied to operational expenses. This suggests that organizations are less likely to make hazard mitigation investments if the **regulatory (non-hazard related) and socio-economic environments impose additional high costs** on the focal organizations.

The situation in which many local government hospitals in large California metropolitan areas find themselves illustrates well the impact of the socio-economic environment. Many county hospitals in California are administered through the local County Departments of Health. In the case of Los Angeles County and the City-County of San Francisco, the county hospitals are affiliated with university medical schools and serve as teaching hospitals. They both provide trauma centers and, because they are public, serve a disproportionately large share of medically indigent and uninsured patients. The hospital administrators report to the heads of the respective Health Departments and, through them, to elected executives and the county board of supervisors.

California's large local government hospitals charge fees for service where practical, but they operate at a loss. Their operations are subsidized through their respective county budgets. Many local government hospital facilities do not meet SB 1953 standards. Hospitals owned by general purpose local governments are at the mercy of the voters and elected local officials who have to make difficult decisions about allocating scarce resources. Finding the capital resources to retrofit or rebuild those large local public acute care hospital facilities is exceptionally difficult. California's state and local governments are experiencing serious financial problems. The State's financial problems over the last two decades are the stuff of legends.

Local governments face taxing and spending restrictions imposed by voters and state government. The need for tax funds to support local activities at reasonable levels of performance far exceeds the supply. Hospitals must compete with all the other public needs for capital investment resources. Los Angeles County received money from the Federal Emergency Management Agency (FEMA) to rebuild its main acute care facility because it was damaged in the 1994 Northridge Earthquake, but, even so, political conflict delayed the construction. San Francisco General Hospital decided early to rebuild its acute care facility, but did not have the money to do so right away. Whether local government hospitals in large urban centers serving the poor will be able to comply with the requirements of SB 1953 without significant outside funding, such as that provided to Los Angeles County by FEMA, remains an open question.

While regulation such as that described in the preceding paragraph might be expected to divert attention away from hazard mitigation investments, other regulations can serve to direct attention toward hazard mitigation investments. Most directly, regulation can compel investment in hazard mitigation. Whether such regulation will cause or help top managers to think in terms of economic benefits and costs is our concern here. Regulations may be written so that they permit a full range of possible hazard mitigation investments, any of which might be expected to yield the desired outcomes of such mitigation (e.g., patient safety in the aftermath of an earthquake). In addition to supporting a wide array of mitigation investments, such regulations may be written with flexible deadlines and approval procedures that recognize the idiosyncratic contexts facing individual hospital organizations. Under these flexible circumstances, we would expect organizations to consider possible hazard mitigation investments in view of their ability to reduce operating or transaction costs, or to permit the charging of higher prices. In general, we believe that organizations are more likely to perceive economic incentives for making hazard mitigation investments if the **implementation flexibility** associated with hazard mitigation regulations is high.

Likewise, regulations may be written so that the cost of not meeting specified hazard mitigation requirements is sufficiently high, perhaps even escalating as time goes by, to attract top management attention. Faced with increasingly high costs for non-compliance, organizations will look for ways to comply as soon as possible, and as cheaply as possible. Since all organizations facing the regulation must comply with it, organizations must rely on both established connections with those who can supply hazard mitigation services (e.g., structural engineering firms) and subsequent speed of compliance to provide any measure of competitive advantage. Organizations that are able to make their hazard mitigation investments quickly while relying on established networks are likely to be rewarded with lower transaction costs (e.g., of construction) than are those organizations that follow. To that end, albeit perhaps only in the short run, such "first-mover" organizations are likely to comply quickly in order to minimize their transaction costs and make the case for higher prices. Thus, organizations are more likely to perceive economic incentives for making hazard mitigation investments if the **costs associated with non-compliance** with hazard mitigation regulations are high.

In order for these costs to have the expected effect, affected organizations must believe that the costs will be applied to them if they fail to comply with the regulation. In other words, simply creating regulations that penalize organizations that fail to comply by a given deadline will not compel cooperation. The organization must believe that the costs (i.e., the future punishment) will actually be administered in order for the costs to influence present behavior (i.e., hazard mitigation). In the case of California hospitals, many of our interviewees told us that they did not believe that the punishment associated with non-compliance with SB 1953 (i.e., loss of licensure) would be meted out, since that would result in fewer acute care hospital facilities being open, the antithesis of the legislation's intended outcome.

One final way in which economic considerations may affect hazard mitigation investment decision-making may be the simplest to understand. Certainly, it is one of the first to be mentioned by hospital executives. In choosing whether to implement various hazard mitigation measures, administrators are likely to develop and weigh a number of financial ratios and financially-oriented considerations. The first among these is often "return on investment." For example, if the hospital organization elects to spend \$30 million on the seismic retrofit of an acute care bed tower, will the organization be able to reclaim any of that investment over the course of the building's remaining lifespan? Or, if the hospital organization decides to spend \$528 million on a new acute care facility, one that uses the latest base isolation technology, will the organization be able to reclaim any of that additional seismic investment over the course of the building's remaining lifespan?

Whether the expenditure makes economic sense depends in part on the probable maximum loss (PML) likely to result from an earthquake or other disastrous event (Woo 2002). Insurers calculate the probability of a maximum credible earthquake (MCE) for given regions and then determine the maximum amount that they are willing to insure. Organizational decision makers must simultaneously weigh several hazard and vulnerability factors in order to make sound economic decisions for their organizations. In addition to considering PML, decision makers must also consider the potential cost of business interruption, the potential loss of revenue and profit, the potential loss of market share, the potential negative impact on the organization's reputation, the potential loss of staff and the need to rehire at possibly higher salaries, and so on. All of these potential costs and losses must be considered in a probabilistic frame, wherein the decision makers assess the likelihood that a damaging earthquake will strike their facility in a given timeframe. Earthquakes don't have seasons like hurricanes do, and the science of earthquakes is such that predicting their occurrence is inexact. Seismologists will say that a geographic area "is due" for an earthquake, but they can't reasonably say when.

On a basic level, hospital administrators must decide which cost will be greater: (1) the cost of seismically retrofitting their existing buildings or building new facilities that are "up to" or exceed seismic building code; or (2) the cost of <u>not</u> seismically retrofitting or building new. The former are costs to be incurred in the near future, with relative certainty as to when and how much. The latter are costs to be incurred in the unknown future, without certainty as to when or how much. We argue that organizations are more likely to perceive economic incentives for making hazard mitigation investments if the expected **costs associated with making hazard mitigation investments** are less than the expected **costs associated with <u>not</u> making hazard mitigation investments** (e.g., the cost of recovery in the event of a disaster).

Our interviews revealed considerable support for the idea that economics was a major driver of hazard mitigation decision making in California hospitals. Executives spoke at length about their hospitals' financial difficulties: historical, current, and anticipated. Access to capital, or the lack thereof, was frequently mentioned as a major obstacle to investing in hazard mitigation, as was the expectation that hospitals could not pay simultaneously for increased staffing and hazard mitigation while receiving smaller reimbursements for services provided. The few hospitals that indicated a strong willingness and intent to invest in hazard mitigation were those that (1) believed that such investments would enhance their ability to compete, either through lowering their costs or by increasing their prices; and (2) had access to needed capital or the means to raise needed capital.

For example, executives associated with one investor-owned hospital spoke directly of the need to rebuild their acute care facility so that they could manage their costs and better serve the needs of patients wanting more contemporary services. These executives decided that rebuilding and modernizing their hospital would enable them to acquire a larger share of the hospital market and thereby reduce their overall costs. Likewise, executives associated with the Mills-Peninsula hospital in Burlingame, California, decided to use the latest base isolation technology in their new hospital, despite increased initial or first costs, in part because they perceived that the life cycle costs would be reduced. The new hospital, scheduled to be finished in early 2011, is expected to be "more efficient and cost-effective" than its predecessor, and "safe in an earthquake up to a magnitude of at least 8.0" (Mills-Peninsula Health Services 2010, para. 1). Importantly, the "new hospital will not only survive an earthquake, it will remain operational with minimal or no damage" (Mills-Peninsula Health Services 2010, para. 13). As stated earlier, the cost associated with business interruption can be extremely high. In the case of Mills-Peninsula, it seems apparent that the hospital's administrators decided that the cost of building new, and building with base isolators, was justified given the potential costs associated with a devastating earthquake event.

Of course, the Mills-Peninsula hospital is located less than two miles from the San Andreas fault. Even people living outside California are familiar with the San Andreas fault and believe that earthquakes are a real – and devastating – possibility. That proximity likely makes the cost projections and hazards and vulnerability analysis easier to believe and act upon.

If any theme dominated our interviews, it was an economic one. In brief: "**No money, no mitigation**."

References

Alesch D, Holly J, Mittler E, Nagy R (2001) Organizations at risk: what happens when small business and not-for-profits encounter natural disasters? Technical report. Public Entity Risk Institute, Fairfax

Barker VL III, Mueller GC (2002) CEO characteristics and firm R&D spending. Manag Sci 48:782–801

Evans JR (1997) Applied production and operations management, 5th edn. West Publishing, St. Paul

Hambrick D, Mason P (1984) Upper echelons: the organization as a reflection of its top managers. Acad Manag Rev 9:193–206

Hertwig R, Barron G, Weber EU, Erev I (2004) Decisions from experience and the effect of rare events in risky choice. Psychol Sci 15(8):534–539

Hess DB, Arendt LA (2006) Critical care in crisis: decision making in New Orleans' hospitals. In: Natural Hazards Center (ed), Learning from catastrophe: quick response research in the wake of Hurricane Katrina, 177–213. Boulder, CO

Katz D, Kahn RL (1978) The social psychology of organizations, 2nd edn. Wiley, New York

Mills-Peninsula Health Services (2010) Earthquake safety. http://www.mills-peninsulanews.org/technology/

Molpus J (November 2004) M.D. or MBA? The two sides of a healthcare CEO. Executive Survival Guide. Retrieved 25 Nov 2005 from: http://www.healthleaders.com/survival/article/60166

Petak WJ, Alesch DJ (2004) Organizational decision making with respect to extreme events: healthcare organizations respond to California's SB 1953. In: Bruneau M (ed) Research progress and accomplishments: 2003–2004 (MCEER-04-SP01), University of Buffalo, State University of New York, Multidisciplinary center for earthquake Engineering Research, Buffalo, NY, May 2004

Porter M (1980) Competitive strategy. Free Press, New York

Sharfman MP, Meo M, Ellington RT (2000) Regulation, business, and sustainable development: the antecedents of environmentally conscious technological innovation. Am Behav Sci 44:277–302

Waller MJ, Huber GP, Glick WH (1995) Functional background as a determinant of executives' selective perception. Acad Manag J 38:943–974

Wiersema MF, Bantel KA (1992) Top management team demography and corporate strategic change. Acad Manag J 35:91–121

Woo G (2002) Natural catastrophe probable maximum loss. British Actuarial Journal, vol. 8 (Part V):943–959

Chapter 11
Organizational Differences in Hazard Mitigation Investment Decision Making: Outside the Organization

In this chapter, we present two additional categories of factors that we believe influence whether, why, and how individual hospital organizations make extreme hazard mitigation investment decisions. Both categories reflect the impact of the external environment on the organization's internal workings and decision-making process.

As with the last chapter, we describe each category from a theoretical perspective, drawing on relevant academic literature. Then, we augment our description of each category with examples drawn from our qualitative research. The extent to which any given hospital relies on these factors to make hazard mitigation decisions is variable and contextual.

11.1 Institutional Predictors

11.1.1 External Institutional Pressures

DiMaggio and Powell (1983) describe three sets of forces that compel firms to behave similarly and appear isomorphic: normative, mimetic, and coercive. We believe that all three forces may play a significant role in influencing hazard mitigation investment decision making.

As described by Sharfman et al. (2000, p. 282), **normative isomorphic forces** "occur when some actor can influence the collective values of a focal firm." Professional associations, especially those to which a focal organization might belong, are most likely to engender such normative forces. Professional associations often craft statements and standards of expected professional conduct on the part of their member organizations and decision makers. Enforcement of such standards often takes an organic form, relying on promises of compliance, publicized expectations for member behavior, and "peer pressure." This contrasts with more bureaucratic forms of enforcement that often include the administration of punitive measures for non-compliance. Thus, for hospital organizations in particular, statements about

D.J. Alesch et al., *Natural Hazard Mitigation Policy: Implementation, Organizational Choice, and Contextual Dynamics*, Environmental Hazards,
DOI 10.1007/978-94-007-2235-4_11, © Springer Science+Business Media B.V. 2012

the value of hazard mitigation investments by state hospital associations (e.g., the California Hospital Association) or national hospital associations (e.g., the American Hospital Association) might reasonably be expected to influence positively such hazard mitigation investment decisions.

In addition to professional associations of which they may be members, organizations may also find themselves influenced by other external organizations and professional associations. In the case of hospitals facing hazard mitigation investment decisions, structural engineering (SE) firms have the potential to be especially influential. SE firms, like all firms, have reputations based on both their firm's prior achievements and on the professional credibility of their principals. If a trusted SE firm advises a hospital organization that it should consider using base isolation for its next new hospital, for example, there is an increased likelihood that the hospital will do so. After all, it would be unusual for a top hospital administrator to be independently familiar with the latest seismic technology. Instead, he or she will rely on trusted colleagues for that information, whether they work in the facilities management area of the hospital organization or for an SE firm.

One non-hospital professional association likely to have some measure of influence on hospital decision making is the association representing the views of structural engineers (e.g., SEAOC – Structural Engineers Association of California). As a group, structural engineers and structural engineering firms are expected to be strong advocates of hazard mitigation, since that is their "bread and butter." The professional associations to which they belong influence heavily what they know and are willing to propose to potential and existing hospital clients.

To the extent that both structural engineering firms and their professional associations are able to make themselves heard by hospital decision makers, and to be found credible in their assertions, we cxpect that they might influence positively the hazard mitigation investment decisions made by hospitals. One of the more challenging aspects of any persuasive attempt is that structural engineers and top managers tend to communicate using different words, reflecting their different perceptions about what matters and reflecting their different functional expertise and education. Where structural engineers might talk of annualized losses, hospital administrators are more likely to be interested in cash flow and return on investment. Where hospital administrators talk about continuity of operations, structural engineers refer to building codes that require life safety and downtime. Hospital administrators involved in multiple building or retrofitting exercises are more likely to understand and appreciate engineering parlance, whereas structural engineers who have worked directly with numerous hospitals are more likely to address life cycle costs. Opportunities to interact and clarify meaning facilitate trust building and persuasive communication.

Within the organization, top administrators may find themselves influenced by the values and demands of the non-management staff members who comprise the organization. These staff members (e.g., nurses, data and lab technicians, food service staff members) may communicate their values and demands individually or through unions or other groups that represent them collectively. The values and demands of these individuals are as likely to be influenced by their profession at least as much as by their interaction with a given hospital. For example, what nurses expect from a given hospital is probably influenced more by the values, needs, and expectations of the nursing profession, relevant unions, and society at large than by what the particular hospital does or says.

In the case of hospitals facing hazard mitigation investment decisions, staff members may perceive that their personal welfare may or may not be improved when the hospital chooses whether to invest in hazard mitigation. Some may believe that the hospital should invest in hazard mitigation in order to protect them and those around them from negative physical consequences in the event of a disaster. Others may believe that the hospital should not invest in hazard mitigation, but instead should offer improved compensation to staff members. What they want will depend greatly on the profession's norms and their personal economic circumstances.

In general, we believe that organizations will respond positively to external normative forces in the sense that they will abide by those forces, to the extent that doing so is economically feasible. In other words, organizations will not behave in ways that they believe will harm them economically, or in ways that are not expected to yield improvements in cost or pricing structures. With this caveat in mind, we suggest that organizations are more likely to make hazard mitigation investments if relevant **external forces** (e.g., their professional associations, structural engineering firms, structural engineering professional associations) **support** hazard mitigation investments.

In the case of California hospitals and SB 1953, the Structural Engineers Association of California (SEAOC) appears committed to ensuring that hospital administrators make appropriate hazard mitigation decisions. Of course, our more cynical readers might argue that SB 1953 is a "full employment act" for structural engineers in California, and then ask, "why should anyone be surprised by structural engineers' support of hazard mitigation?"

Certainly, SB 1953 contributes to the likelihood that some structural engineering firms in California will be in good financial shape for some time. And if only structural engineers supported SB 1953 and its requirement that acute care hospital facilities be upgraded or replaced, then we might be cynical as well. In fact, it isn't just California's structural engineers who support taking the measures needed to make hospital buildings life safe and able to function after a maximum credible earthquake event.

The SEAOC website has made available a publication produced by the California HealthCare Foundation, "Best practices for project management, design, and construction of buildings under OSHPD jurisdiction" (California HealthCare Foundation 2006). The publication is the result of collaborative efforts of several different associations. Specifically, the publication is one output of a task force led by Roger Richter, senior vice president of the California Hospital Association (CHA), supported by the California Society for Healthcare Engineers (CSHE) and in cooperation with OSHPD. The individuals involved in developing and reviewing the publication represent a variety of organizations, including structural engineering firms, architectural firms, hospital organizations (government, non-profit, and investor-owned), the CHA, the CSHE, OSHPD, and several California universities.

It seems reasonable to think that hospital administrators might find useful a "Best practices" document, especially one that had been developed and vetted by a broad array of credible professionals. After all, as the publication states, "California hospital buildings are considered by many architects and engineers to be the most complex buildings in the world to construct. They are also among the most costly" (California HealthCare Foundation 2006, p. vii). The broad and complex array of decision making needed to produce and pay for such buildings is likely made easier by the availability of a source document representing the perspectives of many trusted and knowledgeable colleagues.

In addition to normative forces, mimetic forces are also expected to influence whether and to what extent organizations elect to make hazard mitigation investments. As described by DiMaggio and Powell (1983), **mimetic isomorphic forces** compel organizations in an industry to copy or imitate the behavior of market-leading (first-mover) organizations. The more competitive the industry, the more likely that mimetic forces will induce an observable level of mimicry in behavior and desired outcomes, as organizations pursuing a K-strategy (late entrants) seek to maximize their profits and standing (Brittain and Freeman 1980).

According to the hospital administrators we interviewed, and as described earlier, the hospital industry is considered a highly competitive industry, in part because the competition extends beyond that for patients or end-users. Hospitals compete for administrators, physicians, nurses, and other staff members. Hospitals compete for insurance providers. Hospitals compete for land. Hospitals compete for financial capital. Hospitals compete for philanthropic donations. In many ways, the munificence (Dess and Beard 1984) afforded by hospitals' task environment is low, such that hospitals are constantly competing for hotly contested resources. Without question, the competitive landscape facing hospitals is a hostile one (Covin and Slevin 1989), fraught with the ubiquitous advertising (e.g., billboards, radio, fliers, social media), expensive compensation packages, and donor events that typify competitive industries. To the extent that the leading hospitals in an area choose or do not choose to make and promote hazard mitigation investments, we would expect other hospitals to follow their lead. In fact, we argue that organizations are more likely to make hazard mitigation investments if the perceived **market leaders in the focal industry invest** in hazard mitigation.

The Mills-Peninsula hospital in Burlingame is described as "the first hospital in California to use friction-pendulum bearings" (Mills-Peninsula Newsroom 2011, para. 6), a type of base isolation technology. Widespread innovation diffusion often requires successful and visible testing of the innovation (Kash and Rycroft 2002). In the case of seismic technology, it is likely that base isolation will be adopted by more and more hospital organizations as these organizations observe competitors using the technology, and doing so successfully. Specifically, we expect that a fair number of hospital organizations will implement base isolation technology, which is appropriate for retrofitting or building new structures, if a significant earthquake event occurs in the San Francisco area and the Mills-Peninsula hospital facility emerges "operational with minimal or no damage" (Mill-Peninsula hospital 2010, para. 14) as expected. Late entrants to base isolation will adopt the technology in part because they have seen it work for the first-movers like Mills-Peninsula.

Finally, DiMaggio and Powell (1983) assert that **coercive isomorphic forces** are strongest in industries and organizations that face high levels of government regulation or ownership. Thus, pressure from government is added to the pressure exerted by normative and mimetic forces to compel conformance with desired behaviors and outcomes. In the case of California hospitals, for example, SB 1953 represents a direct attempt to coerce hospital investment in hazard mitigation through the imposition of negative consequences (i.e., loss of licensure) on hospital organizations that fail to retrofit, rebuild, or alter the use of their acute care hospital buildings by specified deadlines. In brief, because California hospitals are required to be licensed by the State, legislators and seismic advocates seem to believe that threatening to non-renew hospitals' licenses will force hospitals to accelerate the replacement or retrofit of their acute care facilities. As it was, hospitals were not replacing their facilities quickly enough for seismic advocates who thought that the threat to patients from earthquakes should have been sufficient by itself to increase hospitals' interest in hazard mitigation investments. With the exception of these advocates, however, apparently few people believed that patients were actually at risk from earthquakes. As numerous hospital executives told us, "No one has died in a hospital from an earthquake since … I can't remember when, if ever." Certainly, no patients had been killed by an earthquake in any of their facilities, or in anybody else's facilities that had the same characteristics as theirs. The 1971 San Fernando earthquake deaths at the two hospitals are considered anomalous by most present-day hospital executives.

To emphasize a key point: The hospital administrators that we interviewed were all quick to highlight their focus on patient safety. We believe that they were sincere in expressing these sentiments. Thus, their concern for patient safety aligns with the concern for patient safety expressed by seismic advocates. The primary difference in perspectives, at least to the extent that we were able to discern, lies in the different parties' assessment of probable risk, to include an assessment of the likely hazard and probable vulnerability. Virtually all of the hospital administrators with whom we spoke believed that their hospitals would withstand a maximum credible earthquake. Sincerely and truly, they did not think that their hospital buildings would injure their patients or staff in a moderate earthquake event (neither in a worst-case earthquake nor in a mild earthquake). Seismic advocates, on the other hand, appear to expect far worse to happen, and soon. Unfortunately, the nature of earthquakes leaves no objective means – to date, at least – for predicting with great certainty when an earthquake will occur and how strong it will be. Thus, the central core of the disagreement between hospital decision makers and seismic safety advocates is irresolvable except through political or persuasive means.

As suggested by this narrative, the actual effect of attempted coercion depends on the *perceptions* of the individuals or organizations being coerced. In talking with various California hospital executives, for example, just as some don't believe that a maximum credible earthquake will occur any time soon, some also don't believe that the proposed sanction of licensure non-renewal would ever come to pass, any more than they believe that their hospital would suffer significant damage from an earthquake, or any more than they believe that their patients would be injured in the event of an earthquake.

Many of the executives we interviewed expressed doubt that the State of California would revoke their acute care license if they failed to comply with SB 1953. Instead, most said that such an action would be counterproductive, and that hospital advocates would argue strenuously on hospitals' and communities' behalf. Most believed that some measure of flexibility would ultimately replace the apparent rigidity of the legislation and its associated regulations. The threat of not having adequate acute care, they stated, was far more salient to critical stakeholders (e.g., the surrounding community) than the threat of an improbable earthquake. For these individuals, then, we would expect the impact of attempted coercion on their behavior or decisions to be negligible. Again, potential punishment must be credible in order to serve as an effective deterrent or motivator of behavior, if in fact it ever serves these purposes well.

This does not mean that SB 1953 has had no impact on hospitals' decisions to retrofit or rebuild. To the contrary, some hospitals have used SB 1953 as a catalyst, an enabler even, of plans that were in the making before SB 1953 or of plans that would have been executed even in the absence of SB 1953. The point is that SB 1953s coercive power is less than some might believe or have expected.

Of course, organizations that receive a significant share of their operating budget from government sources may be especially prone to such coercive forces. After all, they rely on government to provide a substantial portion of the inputs (resources) required to perform their primary function. Without government support, these hospitals cannot imagine continuing their existence. In the case of SB 1953, then, one would expect government owned and operated hospitals to believe that their compliance with SB 1953 was an absolute necessity. As we discovered in our interviews, many government-owned hospitals seemed to believe that they needed to comply with SB 1953, no matter whether they believed that the State would non-renew licenses of non-compliant hospitals and no matter whether they perceived that they had the financial wherewithal to comply. They simply "knew" that they had to comply. Consequently, and because they were convinced that a new hospital would serve their communities, several of the government-owned hospitals used or planned to use SB 1953 as a "catalyst for change." SB 1953 became the state-imposed rule that hospitals had to address, whether they wanted to do so or not, if the affected communities wanted to keep their acute-care hospitals. "We have no choice but to comply with SB 1953" was perceived to be more agreeable to taxpayers and persuasive than "we want to rebuild in order to offer modern medical facilities."

One positive associated with coercive measures taken by the State to ensure cooperation with SB 1953 was the perception of hospital administrators that such legislation "leveled the playing field." In other words, since all hospitals had to comply with the legislation, none should be economically disadvantaged by retrofitting or rebuilding, at least in theory. The goal of many hospitals, it seemed, was to delay action in the hopes that (1) retrofitting or rebuilding might be done at lower cost as technology improved, or (2) that the legislative mandate would be eased over time.

In any case, we suggest that organizations are more likely to make hazard mitigation investments if the **believability** of negative sanctions for non-compliance with hazard mitigation legislation is high. Likewise, we suggest that organizations are more likely to make hazard mitigation investments if the level of **government ownership** of the focal organizations is high.

One case study illustrates the potential effects (or non-effects) of coercive isomorphism on a government-owned hospital. The focal hospital is small and located in a rural area. The population of the area is growing steadily and fairly quickly: Retirees have found the community and are moving there in significant numbers. The hospital is the only acute healthcare facility in the area. It serves a large geographic area with relatively low population density.

This acute care hospital is owned and operated by a single purpose local government. The hospital is governed by a small board elected from the population of the district. Elections to board positions are phased so that board members serve staggered terms. This provides some continuity from year to year, but, at the same time, sometimes inhibits rapid change to meet new circumstances. Competition for board positions varies in intensity, depending on the interest generated by current hospital and healthcare issues in the community. Board members tend not to be healthcare professionals.

The hospital is administered by a CEO who is professionally trained in healthcare administration and who has multi-state experience. Positions reporting to the administrator are also held by professionals, but, since the hospital is small (under 100 beds), it has a small budget, and the balance of the managerial staff does not have advanced academic training. Most of their experience has come on the job.

Even though the hospital is in a relatively small, rural area, it is not a stranger to competition. The chief administrator told us he believes that "people go to the closest hospital *they trust*" (emphasis added by the authors). When residents are not confident in the care they might receive locally, they drive long distances to go to larger facilities. He sees it as his job to ensure that the district hospital is one that people can trust for a wide range of acute care services. The hospital has to maintain a competitive position so that it can survive financially and continue to carry out its mission. Hospital operating costs are covered by a combination of user fees and reimbursements from private insurances and Medicare and Medical, so it is important to ensure that patient volume is sufficient to cover direct and indirect costs. The hospital has the authority to levy a tax on real property within the district, but relies on operating revenue to cover operations. It levies a small annual tax to help with capital expenses associated with maintenance and repair of the facility.

Like most other hospitals, the district suffered hard times in the 1990s as it struggled to maintain financial viability in the face of declining reimbursements and rapidly increasing costs. The district used a combination of managerial innovation, legislative provisions that put them in a more favorable financial position, and cost cutting to remain viable.

When SB 1953 was enacted, the district owned an old hospital facility. The facility did not comply with either SB 1953s structural or nonstructural requirements. Moreover, the facility was too small for the growing population and was inadequate for current medical practice. It had been clear for some time that a new facility was needed to help ensure that residents had confidence in the facility and to meet the needs of a growing and aging population. The primary obstacle to building a new facility in a better location was financial. The facility generated sufficient revenue for routine operations, with its reimbursements and the small property tax that it levied, but the income from operations was clearly inadequate to either replace or retrofit the facility to a point where it would be adequate to serve the community's growing needs.

Administrators and the board framed the challenge of complying with SB 1953 as a chance to replace the dated and inadequate hospital facility. They reasoned that they could use the "unfunded SB 1953 mandate" as a means for replacing the facility. According to the hospital administrator, key decision-makers said, "We can use SB 1953 to pass a referendum to replace the facility. The message to voters could be simple. One might say to voters, 'Look what the State has done to us! Now we have to replace our hospital or we won't have any at all.'" The impetus for the new facility would not be perceived, therefore, as coming from overzealous local hospital personnel trying to improve their situation, but, instead, from regulators in Sacramento. (One of the unintended consequences of mandates is that the legislature or regulating agency may be construed as "the bad guy," regardless of the actual intentions and actions of the legislature or regulating agency.)

The challenge was to get a referendum to build a new hospital on the ballot and, then, to put together a campaign that would result in a positive vote for the new facility. With the help of a community advisory board, the district organization did just that. The referendum passed and a new hospital is being built in a new location. Most of the capital costs for construction will be paid by taxes levied on property owners within the district. The district has to find a way to generate approximately 14% of the costs for the facility and equipment. The staff is working on finding sources for these funds. Some may have to come from the hospital's operating budget. Some may come from charitable contributions. The key, according to the chief administrator, is to come up with the money in such a way as to minimize any adverse effects on the hospital's financial balance sheet. No organization can survive in the long-term if short-term operating balances are consistently and substantially negative.

In summary, unlike some hospitals that viewed SB 1953 as "overkill," this hospital viewed SB 1953 as a valuable mechanism for accomplishing a pre-existing goal. The hospital district was able to use the requirements of SB 1953 as a catalyst to motivate voters to levy a tax on themselves to replace their old, inadequate hospital with a new structure that should meet community needs for some decades to come. This raises a central point: Whether coercion vis-à-vis a legislative mandate will be perceived negatively by the affected party depends, at least in part, on the overall context of the affected party, its goals, and the extent to which the mandate aligns with the party's context and goals.

In looking at the effects of regulations on behavior, it is important to consider not only their coercive nature, but also the direct impact of their deadlines. Importantly, laws and regulations such as SB 1953 may contain a **deadline** after which some negative sanction is imposed for non-compliance. Deadlines within laws may constrict the ability of the regulating agency to enforce and the affected parties to comply with the legislation. As stated earlier, organizations may delay their response to a given regulation or mandate for any number of reasons, not the least of which is lack of available capital or access to needed capital. Some organizations may perceive that waiting to invest in hazard mitigation will be to their advantage, as new technologies may be developed that cost less than today's technologies. Such a "wait-and-see" approach (essentially, a K-strategy) is not unusual for individuals, groups, and organizations – all of which may believe that committing to a given course of action too early will cause them to bear too many of the initial costs of developing innovative technologies (Brittain and Freeman 1980). When deadlines are included within legislation, as they were within SB 1953, the regulatory agency loses much needed flexibility to manage the process of compliance. In other words, regulatory agencies can find themselves in positions of inflexibility, as they are required to implement the legislation within narrowly defined parameters.

In considering the direct effects of deadlines on behavior, we are drawn to research on individual, group, and organizational behavior that suggests that temporal pacing has as much to do with behavior and decisions as do specific events. As described by Gersick (1994, p. 12), with punctuated equilibrium,

> Sometimes consciously, sometimes not, groups select the midpoint (or occasionally another time) as a heuristic milestone and use it like an alarm clock, to help ensure they will move fast enough to finish by their deadlines. In effect, groups allow themselves to persist with opening work patterns until the midpoint. The event of reaching the midpoint – not the completion of a given amount of work – stimulates feelings of urgency and an awareness of the deadline and breaks groups' momentum. Groups feel it is time to move ahead.

In looking at organizations subject to a regulation with a deadline, then, we might expect to see more "action" as the midpoint between the regulation's passage and final deadline is reached. In the case of SB 1953, the initial date that would seem to matter to hospital organizations would be the date that the implementation rules and regulations were published – March 1998. The final deadline for ensuring that all acute care hospital buildings meet current seismic safety standards is 2030. Also relevant to this discussion is the deadline of 2008 by which hospital organizations were to have retrofitted their existing non-compliant acute care hospital buildings. Many hospital organizations have successfully pursued an extension of the 2008 deadline to 2013 or 2015, making 2013 or 2015 the *de facto* retrofit deadline. Based on our research, we believe that organizations are more likely to make hazard mitigation investments as the **deadlines** associated with government-mandated hazard mitigation get closer.

If Gersick's (1994) findings are applicable to the case of California hospitals facing SB 1953, and we think they are, then we should not have been surprised to see limited retrofitting action on the part of hospitals before 2003, the midpoint between the publication of the regulations (1998) and the retrofit deadline (2008). With the *de facto* retrofit deadline shifted to 2013 or 2015, we should not have been surprised to see limited retrofitting action before 2006 or 2008. In fact, as of December, 2006, "about 30% of the SPC-1 floor space has(d) been addressed by large construction projects submitted to OSHPD" (Meade and Kulick 2007, p. 26). Further, we should not be surprised to see limited rebuilding action on the part of hospitals before 2014, the midpoint between the publication of the regulations and the final deadline. In general, as deadlines approach, we expect to see more action on the part of hospitals responding to coercive pressure.

Importantly, the deadline most likely to influence behavior is the one seen as most believable, most achievable, and often, the latest in a series of deadlines. In the case of SB 1953, hospitals' financial condition in the 1990s and into the next decade were poor, making compliance with the earliest deadlines virtually impossible for all but a relatively small number of SPC-1 classified hospitals. Another likely contributor to the minimal compliance with the earliest deadlines would be the unexpectedly high cost of retrofit (Meade and Kulick 2007). By the time a hospital organization completed its costly retrofit, it would have to begin planning for its mandatory 2030 rebuild. Given the high cost of retrofit and the relatively early deadlines associated with retrofit, it seems likely that most hospitals would turn their attention to the latest and the most cost-effective of the deadlines for structures, the 2030 rebuild deadline.

11.1.2 Internal Institutional Pressures

Pressure to make hazard mitigation investment decisions emanates from the inside of organizations at least as much as it emanates from the outside. In particular, aspects of the organization's authority and political structure are likely to influence whether and to what extent the organization invests in hazard mitigation. We include our discussion of internal institutional pressures in our chapter on "the view from outside the organization" in part because institutional theory asserts that organizations act in response to external forces. This is most apparent in a discussion of external institutional pressures but is also relevant to a discussion of internal institutional pressures since the organization's internal workings (structure) enable it to respond effectively to external forces and adapt accordingly.

In general, we suggest that organizations having a more mechanistic structure (Burns and Stalker 1961) will be less likely to invest heavily and proactively in hazard mitigation. Of the elements comprising a mechanistic structure, three are especially likely to hinder proactive and positive hazard mitigation investment decisions: high degrees of centralization, high degrees of formalization, and high complexity in the form of vertical and horizontal differentiation. The overarching purpose of a mechanistic structure is to enable efficiency through a focus on stability and standardized behavior. This contrasts with the purpose of an organic structure, which is to enable responsiveness through a focus on flexibility (Burns and Stalker 1961).

In organizations with a high degree of **centralization**, strategic decisions tend to be introduced by one or a few members of the top management team, i.e., the dominant coalition (Burns and Stalker 1961; Cyert and March 1963; Pugh et al. 1968). Likewise, in organizations with a high degree of centralization, the decision-making platter of the top management team will be relatively full, with many decisions competing to be made. Decisions brought for top-level management consideration tend to result from what Fredrickson (1986, p. 284) calls, "proactive, opportunity-seeking behavior." Since top-level management is the origin or screener of virtually all strategic decisions in a highly centralized organization, it stands to reason that the content of most strategic decisions will reflect the particular interests, functional expertise, and knowledge of an organization's top-level managers. If none of the top-level managers has an interest, background, or other connection to hazard mitigation, then it seems likely that none of them will bring the issue of hazard mitigation investment to the strategic decision table for proactive consideration.

In looking at the particular case of hospitals, it seems likely that few members of top-level management will have achieved their positions through the route of facilities or risk management or emergency preparedness, the functional homes for most hazard mitigation investment decisions. Instead, the hospital executives with whom we have spoken and the individuals involved in final decision making around hazard mitigation tend to have backgrounds and credentials in health administration, business administration (finance), public administration, and medicine. In fact, except in organizations with a mission related directly to facilities management, it seems likely that few top-level managers will have backgrounds and credentials in facilities management or emergency preparedness. To this end, we suggest that top-level managers are less likely to proactively engage in hazard mitigation investment decision making in organizations with **centralized** strategic decision processes.

Our interviews with facilities or risk management and emergency preparedness personnel made clear the importance of the direct link to top management, especially in highly centralized hospital settings. Few top managers were described as being intrinsically interested in hazard mitigation or disaster preparedness. Accordingly, whether such issues made it to the top management decision-making table depended, at least in part, on the hierarchical connection between the facilities or risk managers (emergency preparedness personnel) and members of the top management team. Personnel who reported directly to the CFO or the COO had the best rate of timely success in terms of hazard mitigation requests granted. The further away from the top management team, the more difficult it is to successfully make a hazard mitigation "pitch." Individuals without a direct link to the top management team have to work to establish their credibility and gain space on the top management team's decision-making agenda. Even then, their request may struggle to be considered worthy of the organization's limited resources. Facilities managers, in-house structural engineers, and emergency preparedness personnel tend to constitute a less powerful constituency than doctors, whose equipment needs are both expensive and often revenue-producing (e.g., an MRI machine). Further, their requests are often presented in a negative light, e.g., "We should install an onsite well in order to minimize dependence on a city water source during a disaster," as opposed to the more positive light associated with equipment purchases, e.g., "This equipment will generate X amount of revenue in time period Y, yielding a return period of Z."

A slightly different picture emerges in organizations having a high degree of **formalization**. By definition, these organizations rely on many written rules, regulations, and policies to guide their decision making and activities (Burns and Stalker 1961; Pugh et al. 1968). As described by Fredrickson (1986, p. 284), "the strategic decision process will be initiated only in response to problems or crises that appear in variables that are monitored by the formal system." Unless an organization has a department or similar mechanism charged with monitoring hazard mitigation investments, the organization will not consider them a topic requiring strategic decision making. In the event that an organization does have such a department or similar monitoring mechanism, then we would expect strategic action around hazard mitigation to "be the result of standardized organizational processes" (Fredrickson 1986, p. 284). For example, we would expect hazard mitigation investment decision making to be made in the context of the organization's standard budgeting cycle and process, such that hazard mitigation investment decisions would be subject to the same criteria applied to all potential capital or operating investments. Given the competition for resources within most organizations, it seems likely that most hazard mitigation investment decisions would produce only incremental results (Fredrickson 1986).

Similarly, Sharfman and his colleagues (2000, p. 284) suggest that high degrees of formalization "as characterized by high corporate 'hurdle rates' or inflexible approaches to discounted cash flows" might prove restrictive. While Sharfman et al. (2000) are interested in the particular case of "green innovation," we see their topic as sufficiently analogous to hazard mitigation investments in that both green innovation and hazard mitigation are characterized by less visible and less immediate payoffs. Thus, decision makers considering either green innovation or hazard mitigation often must make their decisions while trusting that they will yield long-term and perhaps socially responsible benefits, benefits that may not be visible until after the current management has moved on.

As described by Sharfman et al. (2000), managers are known to assert that their strategic decision making relies on a rational decision making model that includes financial analysis as its cornerstone. Two financial tools are seen as particularly relevant to innovation decision making, "hurdle rates" and discounted cash flows. Based on our interviews with hospital executives, we believe that these same tools are seen as relevant for hazard mitigation decision making in organizations. In brief, hurdle rates may be defined as the internal return on investment (ROI) targets that capital and other internal investments must meet or exceed in order to be approved by upper-level management. Likewise, discounted cash flows may be defined as the future value of present-day investments. Whether an organization uses either hurdle rates, discounted cash flows, or both, the objective of such financial analysis is to assess the potential capital investment's contribution to "the bottom line." The more formalized the organization and its capital decision making process, the less flexibility we would expect to find in the use of these financial tools. Consequently, it may be difficult for hazard mitigation investments to be approved as part of the usual capital budgeting process, since the timeline for observing effects on profits or costs from hazard mitigation investments may exceed that used in standard discounted cash flow analysis. Complicating this is the reality that many hospitals (and other organizations) tend to set relatively short timeframes (e.g., 18 months) in which to observe positive impacts (e.g., payback).

Additionally, it may be difficult to demonstrate that investing in hazard mitigation will ever have a positive impact on the bottom line, since the costs associated with failing to invest in hazard mitigation may become apparent only if the organization is confronted with a serious hazard. As described earlier, it is no easy task to preemptively calculate the costs associated with an extreme hazard. The cost of closing a hospital, completely or partially, depends on the length of the closure and the ability to conduct operations off-site. Hospitals in New Orleans were exposed to significant costs when they closed after Hurricane Katrina in 2005 and Hurricane Gustav in 2008. Executives at these hospitals told us that their experiences had taught them that closure was an outcome to be avoided at nearly any cost (Hess and Arendt 2006).

The costs associated with staff or patient injury or death depend on the proximal causes and the ability to minimize such injury and death. The cost of a damaged reputation may be incalculable. Who knows which future staff members and patients might avoid a hospital that did not care for its own when needed? Who knows which philanthropists might choose to donate their money and time to other causes? The less probable the particular hazard, the more difficult it may be to show negative cost consequences for lack of hazard mitigation, because the costs are so difficult to quantity in the face of such uncertain parameters.

Based on our research, we argue that organizations with a high level of **formalization** will engage in hazard mitigation investment decision making to the extent that they have a formal mechanism for monitoring hazard mitigation issues (e.g., a facilities management or risk department). The more formalized the strategic decision process in an organization, the less likely that hazard mitigation investment decisions will be easily approved by top-level managers as part of the usual capital budgeting cycle and process.

The following case illustrates how hazard mitigation investment decisions must meet the same criteria as other capital investment decisions in highly formalized organizations, and how they may suffer in comparison.

This non-profit hospital is not associated with any religious organization, but is dedicated to serving what it sees as its community and its market. The hospital has been strained lately because several larger hospitals in adjoining areas have closed. Each of them was in financial trouble before, but "SB 1953 tipped the scale and they had to close." This puts an additional burden on our case hospital, forcing administrators to think seriously about adding capacity.

The dozen or so top administrators at this hospital have uncharacteristically long tenures in their positions. Administrators in California hospitals, especially those in corporations owning numerous facilities, tend to change jobs and locations frequently. Average CEO tenure is typically less than six years. Moving from one corporation to another is commonplace and most administrators have met many of the others in their field as they have relocated from place to place and been promoted from job to job, up the corporate ladder. The administrators at the case hospital are professionally trained in areas such as finance and nursing, and have extensive experience in their areas of expertise. Successful experience means that they tend to use tried-and-true decision methods and criteria.

Like most other California hospitals, this hospital experienced financial difficulties during the 1990s. Good management enabled the hospital to survive that period. The hospital now enjoys a modest operating surplus and has established excellent bond ratings from both Moody's and Standard and Poor. Nonetheless, the hospital has considerable long term capital debt for the new buildings that it has constructed over the past two decades to remain competitive and to meet community demand for its services. There is little room for additional debt load.

Remaining competitive is a central concern. Administrators see trends that are making it increasingly difficult for full service hospitals to compete. Physicians and others are opening facilities designed to provide one or another single service that generates relatively high reimbursements from insurance companies, Medicare, and MediCal. These specialty organizations generate substantial profits for their owners and are essentially unregulated by the State. Full service hospitals are then left to provide the services that pay disproportionately low reimbursements and to comply with high standards imposed by State government. Competition, then, is not just against other full service hospitals, but also against investor-owned organizations seeking to draw off profitable procedures outside the hospital. Under those circumstances, devising effective strategies by which to compete becomes extremely difficult.

The hospital's main acute care building does not comply with SB 1953 structural standards and must be retrofitted, replaced, or withdrawn from service. The hospital needs to have an acute care facility, so it must somehow find a way to comply with the legislation.

The initial estimated cost of retrofitting the acute care building using a standard approach was far in excess of $100 million. Hospital administrators told us, "We don't want to put that much money into a building we will have to vacate in less than 20 years." Thus, the administrators and its governing board have continued to search for a workable, affordable alternative. The design group, which meets every 2 weeks, has sharpened its cost estimates. Even the revised cost estimates have been too high, leading the organization to explore and evaluate alternative approaches, including employing a much less expensive retrofit using new technology. "Economics is driving this. At this point, it is all about survival. Unfortunately, we see no value added by SB 1953. It's just costs we have to absorb without improving our capacity to provide medical care." Hospital administrators feel that their current acute care facility is not at risk from collapse due to an earthquake. Nor are they particularly concerned about the effect of an earthquake on their ability to provide services to victims. "The problem will not be whether hospitals are operable; it will be whether the injured can get to the hospitals."

The preference of this hospital's administrators is to replace the existing acute care facility with a new building, and to convert the existing acute care building to another use, as allowed in the legislation. This preference is driven by the increased demand brought about because neighboring hospitals closed their doors, but also because of administrators' belief that putting money into structural retrofit is a waste. The ROI for a retrofit is not positive. The facility will not be large enough to meet the growing need and is simply money taken away from a new facility. Still, there are some problems associated with building a new facility. "If we have to buy additional land, we have to keep in mind that land here costs more than $50 a square foot." Again, the organization is confronted by the need to achieve a given ROI range for its capital investments, in order to make them worth pursuing. The administrators are also concerned with construction costs that they see as escalating daily, along with long delays waiting for plan approval from OSHPD. "We've looked at a lot of alternatives, but we still don't know exactly what to do. We keep looking at the economics of the situation and trying to decide on the best use of the money we have, given all the things that are needed at the hospital." In this case, hospital administrators were confronted with a seemingly intractable problem. They needed more money than was available to them to do what they really wanted to do (rebuild), and could not countenance spending money on a "temporary fix," a retrofit that would prove cost-prohibitive.

Organizational complexity is a function of both horizontal and vertical differentiation, as well as spatial dispersion (Hage 1965; Fredrickson 1986; Pugh et al. 1968). First, the more departments or functions at a given level in the organization, the more horizontally differentiated is the structure. Next, the more levels in the organization, the more vertically differentiated is the structure. Finally, the more locations that comprise the organization, the more spatially dispersed the structure. Organizational complexity may or may not be related to organizational size, in terms of number of employees or other assets. For our purposes, we focus on horizontal and vertical differentiation alone, since they are primarily responsible for "impos(ing) boundaries of rationality on (organizational) members" (Fredrickson 1986, p. 288). In brief, the more horizontally differentiated the organization, and the more vertically differentiated the organization, the more narrowly will each person's sphere of influence be construed, as delineated by each person's position description, reporting relationship, and departmental affiliation.

In looking at the issue of hazard mitigation investment decision making, it seems likely that in highly complex organizations, hazard mitigation decisions may struggle to rise to the top of the strategic decision making pile, especially if the organization is also highly centralized. As described earlier, in centralized organizations decisions are made at the top rather than being distributed throughout the organization. Without a "hazards mitigation champion" on the top management team, getting a favorable decision on hazard mitigation can be difficult. Maybe even impossible.

When it comes to hazard mitigation, organizational complexity can be a deterrent. Few, if any, organizations have a "hazards mitigation" department. In fact, no one person or department is likely to be responsible for all forms of hazard mitigation, which optimally requires input and "buy-in" from all categories of organizational members. Allocating organizational resources to hazard mitigation requires not allocating resources to other organizational needs, needs that are likely more visible to more stakeholders and more likely to generate revenue (e.g., medical equipment) or decrease costs (e.g., electronic monitoring technology). Hazard mitigation is interdisciplinary and requires collaboration of stakeholders on needs identification and resource allocation.

The more complex the organization, the more unlikely that such "interdisciplinary" concerns will be vetted, except at the organization's top level, which serves as the complex organization's key integrating mechanism. Each department in a complex organization is responsible for a finite and well-defined set of allocation and innovation problems. That finite and well-defined set of problems, coupled with unique values and jargon, contributes to decision making that may not be optimal for the overall organization. This suboptimization or subunit orientation is common in complex organizations.

According to the Carnegie model of decision making (Cyert and March 1963), bounded rationality contributes to most individuals engaging in a localized search for problems and solutions. Put simply, we tend to look in "our own neighborhood" (function, department, division, etc.) for problems, opportunities and solutions. Thus, while facilities or risk management or emergency preparedness personnel are likely to see the importance of at least some hazard mitigation investment decisions, are individuals in other areas of the organization likely to agree with the facilities or emergency preparedness perspective? Probably not, at least not at the expense of their own department's priorities.

In the specific case of hospitals, for example, it seems plausible that physicians might not value hazard mitigation investments in the same way and to the same extent that facilities or risk managers might. After all, and depending on how narrowly a given physician's position is construed, a physician might well argue that money spent on hazard mitigation is money not spent on critical diagnostic or surgical equipment, both of which might be expected to directly affect achievement of the hospital's mission (e.g., providing state-of-the-art healthcare) and its bottom line.

The more complex the organization's structure, the greater the potential for "us vs. them" thinking and decision making, and the lower the potential for critically evaluating less traditional areas of emphasis, such as hazard mitigation. Based on our research, we argue that hazard mitigation investments are less likely to occur in organizations having a **complex** organizational structure.

Interviewees consistently commented on the difficulties associated with explaining and making relevant hazard mitigation issues to hospital personnel whose primary function did not appear to embrace or involve hazard mitigation. Staff positions tend to be narrowly defined, especially in more mechanistic organization structures, and individuals struggle to see how issues outside their immediate functional areas may concern them. the "win-lose" mentality that suffuses much organizational budgeting turns different categories of staff and different departments against one another. Interestingly, the hospitals in Louisiana and Mississippi seemed to have overcome these difficulties to some extent in the wake of Hurricane Katrina. When asked to explain why doctors, nurses, and other staff members were more willing now to serve on mitigation task forces and standing committees than they had been in the past, the consensus was that these individuals had experienced first-hand the need for the hospital to engage in hazard mitigation investments. They saw how their hospitals responded to the disaster, were in fact intimately engaged in their hospitals' response, and recognized now their vested interest in hazard mitigation. They also appeared to have a better understanding of how a lack of hazard mitigation could make their own functions difficult or impossible to perform. If we can say that disasters accomplish anything positive, one example might be people's enhanced understanding of the interdependencies that comprise the organization. People are jolted (perhaps literally) from their safe, discrete havens and forced to see how their role and function must work effectively with other roles and functions in order for the organization to achieve its primary purpose. Just as individuals find their character under stress, so too do organizations discover the value in synergistic behavior.

This discussion leads naturally into a discussion of organizational politics. In addition to their formal authority structures, the **political structures** of organizations are expected to influence whether and to what extent they invest in hazard mitigation. As described by Pfeffer (1981), lack of goal consensus is a key factor that increases organizational reliance on political rather than rational decision making. Since goal consensus is unlikely to be achieved fully in any organization, it seems reasonable to assert that all organizations are characterized by some level of political activity and decision making. The nexus of power in organizations often depends on the historical pattern of resource allocation (Pfeffer and Salancik 1978), such that those with the greatest proportion of resources tend to possess and will continue to possess the greatest amount of *de facto* power, regardless of what the formal organizational chart might suggest in terms of rational-legal authority (Blau and Scott 1962). In matters of planning and budget, as suggested earlier, the divisions of the organization are likely to play a win-lose game of "us vs. them," such that whatever accrues to "us" is denied to "them."

Decisions to invest in hazard mitigation require substantial resources, so substantial in many organizations that the existing structure of resource allocations may need to be significantly altered. Structural alterations may be especially expensive. This will not be the case necessarily, however, if hazard mitigation advocates are already key players in the organization's political structure. In the more likely former case, resources will need to be redirected away from some previously identified array of activities and toward hazard mitigation. The sheer magnitude of the expense associated with hazard mitigation investments implies that any redirection of resources will be away from an equally significant investment or set of investments. In the end, redirection of resources toward hazard mitigation will likely require and yield a shift in either the political structure of affected organizations or the political affiliation of powerful internal stakeholders (e.g., doctors). Importantly, those occupying powerful positions are unlikely to willingly cede their resources, unless they perceive advantages accruing to their divisions in the organization. Hazard mitigation advocates may have to engage in cooptation, preferably the kind that yields hazard mitigation investments that facilitate and do not endanger high quality medical care. Overall, we suggest that hazard mitigation investments will be less likely or at least more difficult in organizations where extant intra-organizational **political structures** direct resources away from hazard mitigation.

Without high levels of external pressure requiring a particular organizational response, the win-lose game of "us vs. them" tends to be an internal one. Within the organization, divisions "battle" each other for resources, "wage campaigns" to acquire positions, and so on. The game changes when the organization perceives a significant threat from outside, one that must be addressed, such as a legislative mandate that hospitals invest substantial capital in hazard mitigation. Then, the organization as a whole becomes the "us," while those responsible for the external threat (e.g., the government agency charged with administering the legislative mandate) may become "them." As described by Sharfman and his colleagues (2000, p. 285), such external pressure:

> … May cause members of the firm to either pull together and forget petty political concerns or try to find innovative ways to respond to the threat. Conditions of an external threat may cause managers to become more interested in the existence of the 'pie' rather than about the size of their particular 'piece'.

External threats increase group or organizational cohesiveness (Staw et al. 1981). On a practical level, organizational members understand that the organization as a whole must survive in order for them to battle internally for resources. To that end, we expect that they will find the means to redistribute resources such that the external threat may be effectively addressed, i.e., the "foe vanquished." In the case of SB 1953, for example, we expect that all hospital employees would see the value in retaining their licensure. Thus, if a critical mass of hospital members believe that "they" (in this case, State government) will take away or non-renew "our" hospital's license for non-compliance with SB 1953, then the hospital members will likely bond together, as "us," in opposition to "them," and will do whatever is needed to retain the license. Another possibility is that employees within the organization will see the external mandate as facilitating their negotiations with management. In California, for example, employees of some unions have argued that hospitals need to comply with SB 1953 as a matter of ensuring employee work safety. This represents a different set of "us" vs. "them" players, but the political strategizing is analogous.

Whether the redistribution of resources is sufficient to compel long-term political behavior change is uncertain, as other factors are more likely to reassert themselves. In the specific case of hospitals, for example, while resources may be redirected to hazard mitigation investments in the relative short-term, the demands of key physicians (for equipment and staffing) are likely to regain political dominance in the long-term. The primary reason for this readjustment lies in the overarching mission of hospital organizations, which is to provide healthcare, and the primary basis for power in hospital organizations, which is the ability to provide healthcare. In other words, no matter the external impetus for hazard mitigation investments, **hazard mitigation is not the primary function or mission of hospitals; healthcare is**. In the end, the primary mission and its representatives will and must hold sway with respect to long-term resource allocation. Hazard mitigation will be funded only as long as it facilitates the primary function. Still, faced with a high degree of perceived external threat around hazard mitigation, a **coalition of internal organizational participants** will likely band together in support of hazard mitigation investments, at least temporarily.

11.2 Regulatory Relationship Predictors

Finally, we address the direct impact of regulation on organizational behavior. Of the five categories of factors expected to influence individual organizational behavior, we believe that regulation may be the least powerful. In the absence of the other four categories of factors, we argue that regulation alone may not compel behavior change, even when failure to comply with a regulation is associated with apparently punitive measures. While regulation has the potential to substantially direct and alter behavior, and to cause action in a particular timeframe, it cannot accomplish much of anything in a vacuum.

The reaction of California hospitals to SB 1953 neatly illustrates this particular reality. While some might assume that the threatened loss of licensure would be sufficient to persuade California hospitals that they need to retrofit or rebuild their acute care hospital buildings, the delayed action or lack of action on the part of many California hospitals contradicts this assumption. Fundamentally, and importantly, most of the leaders of California's acute care hospitals perceive the SB 1953 situation as follows.

They **do not believe** that their patients and staff are at risk from an earthquake, because they do not believe that their facilities are likely to collapse in the event of an earthquake. Why not? They have not personally experienced a hospital collapse, and/or their current hospital facility has not experienced a collapse, and/or no acute care hospital facility similar to theirs or in their relative vicinity has ever experienced a collapse. Briefly, the salience of a given disaster is prerequisite to any action, or even deliberate consideration of any action.

These leaders have undertaken the non-structural repairs required by SB 1953, because they recognize that non-structural damage (e.g., damage to HVAC units, electrical sources, and plumbing) can seriously disrupt hospital operations and make it difficult or impossible to deliver patient care. These repairs made sense in terms of the bottom line and were doable in the timeframe expected.

Still, because hospital leaders do not believe that their hospital structure is at risk from an earthquake, they cannot justify rationally the substantial expenditures associated with structural retrofit or rebuilding.

They cannot afford the base expenditures associated with retrofit followed by rebuilding.

They cannot afford the logistical costs associated with retrofit followed by rebuilding. Especially for hospitals located in urban areas constrained by adjacent residential or commercial buildings, logistical costs – and the decisions they represent – are major hurdles. Imagine a relatively small hospital (fewer than 100 beds) an its parking lot located in a mixed residential and commercial area, with no room to spare. (This isn't a fictional situation; we interviewed at more than one facility matching this description.) It's not possible for the hospital to retrofit; it cannot conform to the rules about noise, vibration, dust, etc. while retrofitting, and would need to close while doing so. This is not a tenable option. The other option, rebuilding, is likewise see as untenable. Without access to more physical space, the hospital would have to build new in the existing parking space (leaving no parking space in an urban area), demolish the existing hospital, and then rebuild the parking space. In the meantime, doctors, nurses, other staff members, and patients may have found other employment or healthcare providers. Logistical issues are real and costly.

Hospitals cannot afford the loss of business and negative stakeholder reaction associated with retrofit followed by rebuilding. Retrofit is exceedingly costly, and since most hospitals will have to rebuild in a short time, it may be perceived as wasteful.

Few structural engineering firms are willing to commit to estimated costs of retrofitting a hospital, since no one really knows how long will be needed or what will need to happen until (re)construction begins.

Finally, and importantly, many of these leaders do not believe that their hospital facility will lose its license if it fails to comply with SB 1953, because they are often the only acute care facility serving their region. They believe that the threatened loss of license is counter to the asserted purpose of SB 1953, which is to keep acute care facilities open before, during, and after an earthquake.

One case that illustrates several of these statements is that of a relatively small urban hospital housed, essentially, in a single building. The building was built before 1973 and does not meet OSHPD standards. The hospital serves a large lower income neighborhood in a metropolitan area. Most of its patients receive MediCal benefits – California's state assistance for the medically indigent. Fewer than 10% of its patients have medical insurance. Patients who come here have few other options for medical treatment without having to travel a considerable distance. When we asked about the hospital mission, the administrator said, "The best description is that this is a bread and butter community hospital."

The hospital is investor-owned, part of a larger corporation that owns hospitals in California and elsewhere. The hospital experienced major net operating losses for more than a decade, and has only recently begun to break even. Unlike many other hospitals, this hospital has not applied for an extension for complying with structural upgrades, hoping instead that legislation would make irrelevant the need to apply for such an extension. Basically, this hospital is hoping that SB 1953 will go away.

As part of its initial evaluation for SB 1953, the hospital concluded that retrofitting the facility would cost in excess of $10 million, would create major logistical problems (since everything is located in one building and the building's lot is surrounded by other businesses), and would offer no potential for increased income to offset the costs. While it may be possible to raise that money under some scenarios (presumably from a new investor-owner), the entire facility would still have to be replaced to meet the 2030 standards. That would cost at least $100 million and achieving the reconstruction is viewed as completely impossible to administrators, given the hospital's assets and income stream.

With hospital ownership in limbo and with income barely matching expenses, hospital administrators have deferred making any decisions about whether and how to comply with the structural requirements of SB 1953. "We have no idea what we could do to meet those requirements. I can't imagine, though, that the State will close hospitals like this. These people have nowhere else to go."

In other words, while the lack of financial resources makes retrofitting or replacing the hospital impossible from an economic perspective, we believe that the most insurmountable obstacle to retrofitting or rebuilding many hospitals may be the top administrators' (1) **not believing** that a devastating earthquake or other extreme event will occur in the near future, and (2) his or her **believing** that the hospital will stay open no matter the seemingly-coercive consequences of not complying with SB 1953. They do not believe in earthquakes (at least not in any bad ones, anytime soon), and they do not believe that any other organization will choose to address the healthcare needs of their particular population (e.g., urban vs. rural, poor, uninsured). And, they reason, a facility that is less-than-perfect seismically is still better than no facility.

This analysis of SB 1953 and organizations' response to it leads to a basic question, "**Can regulation ever compel desired behavior**?" In the case of hazard mitigation investments, we believe that the answer must be "**Yes**," if the regulation has certain characteristics.

For example, the degree to which the regulatory process is **participative** is expected to influence significantly the likelihood of hazard mitigation investment decisions. Consistent with the participative management literature (e.g., Coglianese and Nash 2002; Conroy and Berke 2004; Wagner 1994), involvement in the design of legislation and concomitant regulations may be critical to successful implementation of legislative mandates. Depending on the extent of the participation, we expect that both sides would have the opportunity to describe fully their goals and intentions, along with any perceived obstacles to and facilitators of change. "Advance warning" of likely obstacles should permit the inclusion of appropriate palliative measures. For example, involving even more hospital organizations in the development of hazard mitigation legislation such as SB 1953 may have given those organizations greater insight into the rationale behind the legislation, while also providing a more realistic view of the organizations and their capabilities to those responsible for crafting the legislation. In the case of California hospitals facing SB 1953, their lack of financial capacity has been a major obstacle in need of attention. While proponents of SB 1953 saw the need to include the means for financial support to the hospitals, the final version included no such provision.

Ideally, the parties involved will display high levels of both cooperativeness and assertiveness, the two ingredients necessary for collaborative problem solving and conflict management (Ruble and Thomas 1976). Cooperativeness focuses on the other party's concerns, and assertiveness focuses on one's own concerns. Whereas the level of cooperativeness indicates the importance of the relationship between the two parties, the level of assertiveness conveys the importance of the issue. High levels of both cooperativeness and assertiveness advance the relevant issues without sacrificing or downplaying the significance of the relationship. The ultimate outcome of collaborative conflict management is problem resolution. In other words, the problem and its root cause(s) are likely to be fully addressed. Likewise, both parties are more likely to be committed to the chosen solution, and more likely to be satisfied that they have been treated fairly.

In the case of SB 1953, it must be emphasized that the hospital organizations alone are expected to bear the financial cost of compliance with SB 1953. In other words, SB 1953 is an "unfunded mandate." While some might argue that the hospitals should be solely responsible for implementing SB 1953 because the benefits of hazard mitigation accrue to them (e.g., remaining functional and continuing to make money after an extreme hazard event), we believe that the logic underlying this argument is faulty.

First, the stated rationale for SB 1953 is the state's desire to keep acute care hospital facilities open in the event of an extreme hazard, in order to serve the larger community.

Hence, the purpose of SB 1953 is to serve the public good, not to ensure that hospitals are able to continue earning revenue. Second, and as previously described, hazard mitigation seldom results in benefits visible to critical stakeholders, must typically be linked with other projects or with other purposes to be financially and politically appealing, and reallocates resources away from other investments that would be more visible and that could be correlated directly with the organization's "bottom line" (e.g., the acquisition of diagnostic equipment). Together, these statements suggest that hazard mitigation by hospital organizations, especially expensive structural hazard mitigation, is a "public good." If the public benefits from the hazard mitigation, such that the public's needs are the driving force behind the mitigation, then we believe that the public should share in the costs of such mitigation. Assigning costs to the current users of the hospital (required when the public does not contribute to paying for hazard mitigation) unfairly punishes those individuals for benefits that will be distributed to any member of the public in the event of an extreme hazard, regardless of their previous affiliation with the hospital entity.

The bottom line? We suggest that organizations are more likely to make hazard mitigation investments if the regulatory process is **participatory**. Further, organizations are more likely to make hazard mitigation investments if the concerns of implementing organizations are **acknowledged explicitly** in the regulatory process and **provisions are made to alleviate the burdens** associated with implementation (e.g., lack of financial capacity).

Whether California hospitals were involved to a satisfactory degree in the development of SB 1953 and the subsequent administrative regulations is debatable. While many individuals perceive that hospital input was solicited and taken seriously, others disagree.

Even if we could transport ourselves back in time, it's unlikely that we could conclusively determine the extent to which the hospitals were involved in the decision-making processes undertaken by the legislature and OSHPD. One person says, "plenty," another person says, "somewhat," and yet another person says, "not at all." Who's right?

In fact, we suspect that all three perspectives are accurate. It's clear that several hospital organizations and the California Hospital Association were involved in the dialogue that yielded SB 1953 and the subsequent administrative regulations. It's also clear that many hospital organizations believed that their concerns went unheard, by both the legislature and OSHPD. Finally, it's clear that some hospital organizations were not involved in any of the decision making.

The first group, those who perceive themselves to have been involved in the decision making, tend to describe the legislation as "understandable" and "not inappropriate." The legislation "levels the playing field," and ensures that all acute-care hospitals will neither collapse nor kill people in a maximum credible earthquake. No one wants to be responsible for failing to protect patients, staff, and visitors. Members of the first group see value in collaborating and working with OSHPD to resolve issues that arose as the regulations were developed and implemented, such as the high number of buildings classified as SPC-1.

The second group, those who believe that their input was solicited but not necessarily taken seriously, tend to be accepting of the legislation, but not of the administrative regulations. They do not hold OSHPD in high regard. They acknowledge that the California Hospital Association has been involved in attempting to address their concerns, but are not particularly hopeful that their concerns will be adequately addressed. During our interviews these individuals complained heartily about OSHPD's apparent lack of responsiveness and speed, and about how it was costing them increasing amounts to comply with SB 1953 as a result.

The third group, those who do not think they were involved at all in the decision-making process, did not think SB 1953 was either useful or appropriate. In fact, when told that the interview's focus was SB 1953, nearly the first phrase uttered by every hospital executive in this group was "unfunded mandate," followed by expressions and gestures of disgust and dissatisfaction. Hospital executives were clear in their belief that those responsible for crafting and implementing SB 1953 did not understand and did not care about the economic situation faced by most California hospitals. Instead, hospital executives shared their belief that legislators had been misled in their quest to enhance access to acute care hospitals by seismic safety advocates who pushed for implementation of the same seismic mitigation measures in all California hospitals, regardless of their actual risk profile and no matter the health of their balance sheet. Since they were not consulted in advance of the legislation's passage, they recognized that current complaints and laments sounded more like "sour grapes" than useful feedback. Many of these executives questioned us as much as we questioned them. "Why can't they just tie seismic upgrades to other remodeling projects, similar to what happens with ADA?" "Why can't they limit their interest to new buildings?" "Why can't they understand that we don't have the money (or the land, or the ability to shuffle patients while we do a retrofit)?"

One case illustrates this last perspective particularly well.

Like 85% of California hospitals, this investor-owned facility suffered net operating losses throughout the second half of the 1990s. It now has a modest operating surplus – three or four points above break-even. The hospital is still struggling to help ensure its continuing financial viability in the face of continuing changes in the industry and in state regulations.

The administrators at this hospital facility think that SB 1953 is bad policy. They described it as a knee-jerk reaction to the Northridge Earthquake of 1994. To paraphrase them, "It's overkill. If the state is really concerned about providing acute care after an earthquake, why don't they consider other alternatives, like field hospitals? This just isn't a cost-effective approach. There is no value added by SB 1953." Further, they are of the mind that, "Without economic and legislative relief, there will be a serious loss of needed capacity" as hospitals close or are converted from acute care to other uses. "Hospitals have closed," they told us, "because owners went through the analysis and said 'there is no way to get from here to there.'" The administrators added that California hospitals were closing because of a whole bundle of events: Staffing problems and state staffing mandates, inadequate reimbursements by government and insurers, the extremely high costs of seismic upgrading, and the "big hospital financial bust" of the late 1990s.

Compliance with SB 1953s structural requirements is "just one more thing in a constant stream of challenges, problems, and change." Administrators said that they have been able to cope with regulations like ADA (improved access for the physically handicapped) and required upgrades for fire protection, despite the high costs of compliance, because of the way the requirements were imposed (e.g., comply when undertaking any major reconstruction), but that the cost of seismic upgrading "is the elephant that is loose in the back room."

The administrators told us that the basic problem is financial. "You can't retrofit or rebuild if you are losing money or just breaking even." Relatively few California hospitals have the capacity to service large capital debt, even if they had the ability to borrow the funds required to replace their noncompliant facilities.

Decision makers in this system determined that it did not make sense to retrofit the acute care facility to meet SB 1953s structural requirements. Retrofit is expensive, takes a long time, and, then, would only extend the life of the building for about 20 years. Replacement is much more sensible. Unfortunately, hospital construction costs are skyrocketing upward.

Administrators at this and other hospitals cited reviews at OSHPD that take two years or more. The cost of structural steel has escalated rapidly to extraordinary levels. Concrete costs are rising at nearly similar rates. "What used to be a cost of about a million dollars a bed is starting to look more like two million dollars a bed," the administrator sighed.

Corporate and facility decision makers are still devising and evaluating alternative means for complying with SB 1953. "We're on alternative 59," they told us, "And we still don't have one that works." The decision process involves the CEO, CFO, Business Development officer, and COO, along with land planners, architects, and the owners – "on particular issues." The corporation's basic intent is to stay in business and to serve the community. As the decision makers continue their search for a viable alternative, they hope for legislative relief.

Looking at all three groups of hospital administrators, there appears to be a continuum of participation in the legislative and regulatory decision-making processes. Accordingly, there appears to be a continuum of perceptions about the "appropriateness" of: the legislation, the regulations, OSHPD, the assessment of buildings (SPC-1, etc.), the proscribed timeline, and so on. While members in each group may be tempted to describe their perception as the "reality," in fact there are many different realities – at least three.

Despite differences in perceptions, most people agree that the legislation and the subsequent regulations may have been written too deterministically, without remedy for changing conditions and without administrative flexibility. Most people also agree that the cost of retrofitting or rebuilding virtually all of California's acute-care floor space cannot be accomplished within a short timeframe, not without incurring unintended and negative consequences such as hospital closures. Finally, most people also agree that the cost should not be borne solely by the affected hospitals, but somehow shared with the communities in which these hospitals exist. Hospitals, after all, serve a public purpose, regardless of their ownership type.

Since our goal is to understand different hospitals' responses to SB 1953, it is critical to understand different hospitals' perceptions. What one perceives becomes one's reality; one's perceived reality is what drives one's behavior.

Importantly, and as described in earlier chapters, many of the issues raised by hospitals have been at least partially addressed. For example, the rating of hospitals as SPC-1 has been reviewed, and fewer hospitals are now in the "worst case" classification. That change alone should ease some of the economic pressure placed on California hospitals. Not yet addressed is a financial means of supporting the hospitals as they undertake the expensive task of rebuilding their acute care hospitals. It's also important to remember that some hospitals, especially those that are better off financially, have used SB 1953 to help them satisfy strategic growth and market competitiveness goals. The consequences of SB 1953 are a mixed bag, depending on each hospital's context and goals.

Whether and to what extent hospitals invest in hazard mitigation measures depends on many factors. The process of hazard mitigation investment decision making is complicated, and its outcomes are difficult to predict. Our goal in developing the preceding theoretical framework has been to suggest plausible explanations for why hospital organizations, like those in California, might choose to invest in hazard mitigation. That hospitals respond differently to the hazard mitigation investment decision lends support to our broadest assertion, which is that hospital organizations do **not** perceive their circumstances, including the imposition of legislation such as SB 1953, similarly. Consequently, they do not respond similarly. They do not make the same choices. They do not weigh the various factors similarly, across factors or hospitals.

One factor that does not appear to reliably determine whether hospital organizations will invest in hazard mitigation is organizational type. Specifically, our research suggests that hospital type (i.e., for profit – private, investor-owned, not-for-profit, or government owned and operated – district hospitals, city/county hospitals and state/academic hospitals) does not, in and of itself, significantly influence whether and to what extent a hospital organization chooses to make hazard mitigation investments. All of the hospital types, regardless of their ownership structure and legal affiliation, must generate revenue in order to maintain and grow their operations. Thus, the **relative financial health** of the overall organization appears more influential than organizational type. More than one administrator confirmed that their hospital organization was expected to generate revenue, to break even, in addition to achieving their mission of serving the surrounding community and providing patient care.

While administrators of the different types of hospitals often commented that other types of hospitals probably made decisions using different criteria than they did, in our interviews we heard the same criteria being used, regardless of organizational type. For example, administrators of non-profit and government-owned hospital organizations often commented that their mission of serving the surrounding community drove their decision making, "unlike what happens at our for-profit competitors." In contrast, the heads of for-profit hospital organizations were as likely to mention their mission of service as often as did the heads of the non-profit and government-owned hospital organizations. As the head of one particular for-profit hospital organization that we interviewed stated, "We see our facilities as having the characteristics of a typical community hospital. Our organization is committed to doing business in and providing service to specific geographically defined communities." All of the administrators conceded that making adequate money was an important goal for their hospital, regardless of organizational type. As much as the different administrators wanted to believe that they thought and acted differently than did their competitors, in fact they acted more similarly than differently, at least with respect to their mission of service. They may weigh factors differently, but they still tend to consider the same or similar factors.

References

Blau PM, Scott WR (1962) Formal organizations: a comparative approach. Chandler Publishing, San Francisco

Brittain JW, Freeman JH (1980) Organizational proliferation and density dependent selection. In: Kimberly JR, Miles RH, Associates (eds), The organizational life cycle, Jossey-Bass, San Francisco, pp 291–338

Burns T, Stalker GM (1961) The management of innovation. Tavistock, London

California Healthcare Foundation (2006) Project management, design, and construction of buildings under OSHPD jurisdiction. Oakland, CA

Coglianese C, Nash J (2002) Policy options for improving environmental management in the private sector. Environment 44:11–23

Conroy MM, Berke PR (2004) What makes a good sustainable development plan? An analysis of factors that influence principles of sustainable development. Environ Plann A 36:1381–1396

Covin JG, Slevin DP (1989) Strategic management of small firms in hostile and benign environments. Strat Manag J 10:75–87

Cyert RM, March JG (1963) A behavioral theory of the firm. Prentice-Hall, Englewood Cliffs

Dess GG, Beard DW (1984) Dimensions of organizational task environments. Adm Sci Q 29:52–73

DiMaggio PJ, Powell WW (1983) The iron cage revisited: institutional isomorphism and collective rationality in the organizational field. Am Sociol Rev 48:147–160

Fredrickson JW (1986) The strategic decision process and organizational structure. Acad Manage Rev 11:280–297

Gersick CJG (1994) Pacing strategic change: the case of a new venture. Acad Manage J 37:9–45

Hage J (1965) An axiomatic theory of organizations. Adm Sci Q 10:289–320

Hess DB, Arendt LA (2006) Critical care in crisis: decision making in New Orleans' hospitals. In: Natural Hazards Center (ed), Learning from catastrophe: quick response research in the wake of Hurricane Katrina, 177–213. Boulder, CO

Kash DE, Rycroft R (2002) Emerging patterns of complex technological innovation. Technol Forecast Soc Change 69(6):581–606

Meade C, Kulick J (2007) SB 1953 and the challenge of hospital seismic safety in California. California HealthCare Foundation, Oakland

Mills-Peninsula Health Services (2010) Earthquake safety. http://www.mills-peninsulanews.org/technology/

Mills-Peninsula Newsroom (2011) http://www.mills-peninsulanews.org/technology/

Pfeffer J, Salancik G (1978) The external control of organizations. Pittman, Boston

Pfeffer J (1981) Power in organizations. Pittman, Marshfield

Pugh DS, Hickson DJ, Hinings CR, Turner C (1968) Dimensions of organizational structure. Adm Sci Q 13:65–105

Ruble T, Thomas K (1976) Support for a two-dimensional model of conflict behavior. Organ Behav Hum Perform 16:143–155

Sharfman MP, Meo M, Ellington RT (2000) Regulation, business, and sustainable development: the antecedents of environmentally conscious technological innovation. Am Behav Sci 44:277–302

Staw BM, Sandelands LE, Dutton JE (1981) Threat rigidity effects in organizational behavior: a multilevel analysis. Adm Sci Q 26:501–524

Wagner JA III (1994) Participation's effects on performance and satisfaction: a reconsideration of research evidence. Acad Manage Rev 19:312–330

Part IV
Beyond the Usual Suspects: Public Policy Design and Contextual Dynamics

Part IV examines the impact that problem framing and policy design have on program implementation, particularly in a dynamic and not-very-predictable socio-economic context. It is critical that policies be designed so that they can be adjusted as dramatic changes occur in the relevant economic environment of both the government that initiated the policy and those who are expected to comply with the policy.

Chapter 12
Mindsets, Policy Design, Congruence, and Related Obstacles to Policy Implementation

12.1 Obstacles to Implementing SB 1953

One should never assume that policy implementation will not encounter obstacles. We have concluded that, if potential obstacles to implementation can be anticipated, steps may be taken to reduce the extent to which they will affect implementation adversely. The obstacles to implementation that plague SB 1953 occur frequently and persistently in the realm of public sector policy-making and program design. Some lessons seem to never quite take hold or to be forgotten periodically.

From our analysis of the SB 1953 experience, we identified three significant obstacles to implementation. To the best of our knowledge, they have not been explored extensively in the scholarly literature on implementation. The first of these is *how the problem is framed* by those who bring it forward as a candidate for public policy action. It seems that, over and over, problems are framed inappropriately or, at least, in a way such that many of those involved in it or affected by it do not fully concur. Ensuring that the problem is framed in a way that is congruent with the mindset of those who are expected to bear the costs of taking the steps necessary to address the problem seems to us to be central.

A second potential obstacle is *the solution approach embodied in the policy* that is intended to address that problem. The solution selected for addressing the problem must be based on causal relationships that hold up under scrutiny and in light of the realities of the system at which it is directed. It seems to us that policies are often formulated as though the authors were absolutely convinced that "If I do x, then y (and nothing else) will happen." We are, or should be, sufficiently sophisticated to understand the extent to which chance events affect even the best laid plans of mice and men. The unanticipated always happens: this has been true since long before Murphy formulated his law.

The third set of potential implementation obstacles is *the context within which implementation takes place.* Dynamic contexts, evolutionary or revolutionary changes or problems, and the emergence of unanticipated consequences during

D.J. Alesch et al., *Natural Hazard Mitigation Policy: Implementation, Organizational Choice, and Contextual Dynamics*, Environmental Hazards,
DOI 10.1007/978-94-007-2235-4_12,

implementation require agile adaptation by government if policies and programs are to stay on track toward goal attainment. California State government was slow to respond to serious and apparent problems that emerged in the first years of implementing SB 1953. Indeed, the legislative and executive branches left it almost entirely to the implementing agency, OSHPD, to find a way – eventually adapting HAZUS to its needs – to make a major adaptation making successful implementation at least plausible.

Here, we explore the first two of the obstacles we found to be particularly important in the SB 1953 experience. We think they are applicable to natural hazard policy generally. For each obstacle, we identify and explore factors we think exacerbate the extent to which each of the potential obstacles becomes an actual obstacle. The third set of obstacles, the context within which implementation takes place, is explored in a subsequent chapter.

12.2 Problem Framing as an Obstacle to Implementation

12.2.1 A Problem from Whose Perspective?

Russell Ackoff (1974) advised that "Successful problem solving requires finding the right solution to the right problem. We fail more often because we solve the wrong problem than because we get the wrong solution to the right problem" (p. 8). This is sage advice. Questions arise, though, as to how we are to know whether we are addressing the right problem.

In the case of SB 1953, the problem was defined for seismic safety advocates by Karl Steinbrugge almost a quarter century before the law was enacted.

> Surely public interest is much better served if hospital structures are designed with sufficient damage control features so as to remain functional after an event. This means not only placing severe limits on permissible structural damage, but also severe limits on permissible elevator damage, telephone and other communications damage, standby power damage and the like (Steinbrugge et al. 1971, p. 56).

Steinbrugge was a well-known and highly respected professor of structural design at the University of California, Berkeley. He served as the first Chairperson of the California State Seismic Safety Commission and as President of the Earthquake Engineering Research Institute. His description of the problem appears to have commanded considerable attention and has had a lasting impact over the years.

From the standpoint of seismic safety advocates, Steinbrugge's was a clear statement of the right problem. They had been working generally systematically through a list of hazardous kinds of infrastructure and facilities to ensure that they were retrofitted or replaced: highway overpasses, bridges, utility lines, etc. Hospitals appear to have been the next on the list. From the seismic safety standpoint, it made sense.

The question is whether the problem might have been framed differently to help ensure that it would make sense to people other than seismic safety advocates. From that standpoint, the problem as formulated had several shortcomings. First, it addressed safety only for those patients and staff members in *acute care* hospitals. Should not the patients and staff in outpatient clinics, chronic care facilities, psychiatric facilities, and other nonacute care facilities be assured the same level of seismic safety as those in acute care facilities? Aren't these facilities also needed after a disaster? In New Orleans, for example, after Hurricane Katrina, health care officials lamented that a dearth of psychiatric care availability was most problematic.

Second, from the standpoint of seismic safety advocates, both the problem and its solution lies in their concern that acute care facilities should be operational following a damaging earthquake to provide assistance to those who have suffered injury from the earthquake. This concern, too, raises questions. Are the victims of earthquakes more worthy of having an acute care hospital available in the aftermath than the thousands who would presumably need such help following a major failure of a levy in the Sacramento area? Certainly, devastating floods are almost a certainty in that locale at some time. After all, there are only two kinds of levees: those that have failed and those that are going to.

Finally, a damaging earthquake is likely to create serious problems for getting people to acute care hospitals because of blocked streets, fires, congestion, and the like. If one were concerned about getting urgent care to those in desperate need, wouldn't one think about bringing portable facilities to the most heavily damaged areas rather than attempting to transport those patients across rubble strewn streets and damaged highways?

At the same time as one might contemplate these questions, it might also make sense to contemplate the problems hospital owners themselves faced because they owned and operated old, generally out-dated hospital facilities. Like California, the States of Washington and Oregon are subject to major seismicity, but they have not enacted legislation similar to SB 1953. Those states simply require that a hospital facility, if it is to undergo substantial modification or replacement, be brought up to contemporary seismic standards. If that pace is too slow for Californians, then ways might have been devised to encourage and facilitate replacing old hospital facilities that are designed for medical practice that is a quarter century out of date. From that perspective, it doesn't make sense to retrofit an old, inefficient hospital facility so that it is an old, inefficient, seismically safe hospital. Doing so would seem to be a significant waste of capital in an industry that, at the time of enactment, was already seriously short of capital.

Here's the main point. The problem might have been framed to accomplish the twin goals of enhancing seismic safety and building an inventory of new, more efficient hospital facilities and a network of hospitals that better met the needs of Californians, hospital owners, and seismic safety advocates. If the problem had been framed from a broader perspective it may well have generated support from a broader base. Not many people in their right mind are against enhancing the seismic safety in hospitals in areas subject to frequent earthquakes. Yet, at the time this is being written, *no one* has died in a California hospital as a consequence of an earthquake since the collapse of the unreinforced masonry Veterans Administration Hospital at San Fernando in 1971, where 49 people died and the death of one person in the collapse of a portico for ambulances at the newly constructed Olive View Hospital in Sylmar.[1] Other health care issues exist in California that are perceived, at least by some people, to have a higher priority than seismic safety and hospitals remaining operational in the immediate aftermath of an earthquake. Many more people die in California hospitals because of preventable medical injuries than because a hospital collapsed on them or because they were unable to get urgent care before they expired. Nationally, "Experts estimate that a staggering 98,000 people die from preventable medical errors each year. More Americans die each month of preventable medical injuries than died in the terrorist attacks of Sept. 11, 2001" (Crowley and Nalder 2009). Why, if preventable medical errors cause so many more deaths in hospitals than do earthquakes, would a state government choose to have hospital owners spend what is now estimated to be $160 billion on hospital retrofit and rebuilding to make hospitals more seismically resistant and do virtually nothing to reduce the number of preventable deaths in hospitals? Why would the state not ensure that a similar amount of money would be spent to ensure that quality healthcare is accessible to all Californians, thus preventing thousands of needless deaths per year?

We are not arguing against enhanced seismic safety; we encourage and applaud it. Nonetheless, it appears to us that the typical array of implementation problems has been exacerbated in connection with SB 1953 because of an overly narrow definition of the "old hospital" problem. Had the problem been framed more broadly to address a variety of issues and interests, it would likely have been more congruent with the hospitals' prerequisites for action. The criteria established to rank hospitals in terms of the urgency with which they were to be retrofit, replaced, or taken from service led to the designation of an extraordinarily large number of facilities as a threat to life and subject to failure. Those criteria were adjusted dramatically years later when OSHPD took the bold move of shifting to a new methodology (HAZUS) to classify hospital facilities needing urgent action and have presented a challenge that is much more tractable.

12.2.2 Problem Framing

Policies are the result of how policy makers and those who have the greatest influence on them make sense of their experience, frame problems, and select a solution intended to address the problem. How the problem is perceived and the basic solution incorporated into the policy makes a difference in how successfully the policy can be implemented and the extent to which it results in desired or inadvertent outcomes. Policy flows from how the problem is perceived and framed, the underlying causal model adopted by the framers, and the intervention/solution selected.

[1]Some will argue that a heart attack death in a hospital damaged by the Northridge Earthquake constitutes a death as a consequence of an earthquake, but such a death may have occurred regardless of whether the individual was hospitalized at the time.

We think the likelihood of successful implementation depends on the extent to which all those involved in the implementation network have shared perceptions of existing conditions, have compatible perceptions of desirable end-states, and generally agree on the appropriateness of the means for achieving the desired end-state. The likelihood of complete concurrence, however, is extremely low. One would certainly expect divergence in goals and perceptions among levels of government, but one would also expect that government officials might have different motives and evaluative criteria than those of organizations whose behavior they are attempting to regulate. Still, if everyone is in general agreement about the ends and the means, successful implementation should be more likely than if there is considerable disagreement about the ends and the means.

We believe that if all the stakeholders concerned with a problem are in general agreement about the nature of the problem and appropriate ends and means, successful implementation is more likely than if there is disagreement about those things. It is, however, rare when all those involved agree on what the problem is or even whether a problem of any consequence exists. If there is little agreement on how the problem is framed, then agreement about ends and means seems unlikely.

The starting point for discussing barriers to implementation is to consider how perceived problems give rise to the policy under consideration. Problems are best seen as disparities between what is desired and what is perceived as reality or pending reality. It is a serious mistake to assume that, because a phenomenon is a problem for you, it is also a problem for everyone else. It is also a serious mistake to assume that, since others do not see things the way you do, they are living in ignorance, not grasping reality, or malevolently inclined.

Petak and Atkisson (1982) state that "the public policy process begins when some state of affairs is perceived as being intrinsically or instrumentally unsatisfactory by an element of society and is perceived by it to qualify as a public problem." Alas, it is often difficult for the actors concerned with policy making to reach agreement on an unambiguous statement of any important problem. First, people do not always share the same perceptions of what is or of what is likely to be. Second, people do not all have the same desires, nor do we place equal value on various possible states of affairs. Third, people do not always share a common understanding of causal relationships. Fourth, in most cases, people are forced to employ subjective estimates of probabilities concerning the distribution of possible outcomes resulting from a set of conditions; those subjective probability estimates range widely. Consequently, it is difficult to achieve agreement among a critical mass of actors concerning problem definition. It is equally difficult to maintain that critical mass over time, especially as conditions and perceptions change.

Harold Lasswell contributed genuine insight into the difficulties in obtaining agreement on ends and means when he elaborated his theory concerning human rationality to different value bases (Lasswell 1976). Lasswell argues that "rationality" in decision making should be judged in terms of the "base" to which one is rational. Not everyone, he suggests, is rational "to the base economic efficiency." Politicians, he says, are more rational to the base "power." That is, they have a tendency to evaluate alternatives, not in terms of economic efficiency, but in terms of how many votes each of the alternatives is likely to garner for them. Urban planners might be rational to a base of "civic beauty and order," and clerics might be rational to a base of "rectitude" by which they would evaluate alternatives in terms of how they squared up with what they perceive to be right in terms of God's law. And, heaven help us, professors may actually be rational to the base "punditry." None of us, of course, is rational to only one value base; we are individually rational to a unique blend of rationalities. Lasswell's construction helps us understand why it is so difficult to get agreement on a statement of the problem: the situation, hence the problem, looks different to each of those peering at it through the lens of their respective mix of value bases.

Lasswell is not alone in his observations. Earlier, Kenneth Arrow (1951) demonstrated the concept in his General Possibility Theorem, better known as Arrow's Impossibility Theorem. Arrow addressed questions of social choice and individual values and preferences. In essence, it is extraordinarily unlikely that any collective policy decision will satisfy everyone because we don't share the same mix of preferences. Problem definition and policy design would be so much easier if, like ants or bees in a hive, we all shared identical concerns and mindsets. Failing that, problems are framed and policies are made depending on who has the most votes or, more cynically, on whose votes count and on who counts the votes.

Conflict about problem perceptions and policy choices is inevitable: what distinguishes societies from one another is how they deal with that conflict. Thoughtful analysis and sensible compromise and accommodation, unfortunately, are relatively rare, at least when fundamental ideological differences exist between those attempting to address an issue or when those who expect to benefit are not those who are expected to bear the costs.

One way to view problem perception is through an analogy. We think of those concerned with a problematic set of phenomena as peering through one of many blurred facets of a cloudy crystal. The crystal is clouded by complexity, uncertainty about causal relationships and the outcomes of intervention, and an array of chance events. The facets are "windows" blurred by our own limitations that hinder clear vision. We peer through the windows in an attempt to make sense of the phenomenon so we can ascertain whether it constitutes a problem for us and, if so, to visualize how best to deal with it. Those with similar values and perceptions tend to group together to peer through only one or two facets.

One might walk around the entire crystal, peering into each facet in a sincere attempt to see what the phenomenon looks like through each of the many facets. Presumably, doing so might enable one to make sense of the situation from several perspectives, identifying the critical perceptual differences that exist between those who choose to look through only one or two facets. As it turns out, though, phenomena that are candidates to become public problems leading to some form of government action are usually championed by an interest group dominated by a particular mindset. In the case of SB 1953, the cluster of interested parties initiating the concern was dominated by those with a special concern about employing seismically resistant buildings to enhance seismic safety. Their primary concern with hospitals appears to be that they would be able to function after an earthquake to treat the injured.

They do not appear to have been especially concerned about all the other functions that hospitals perform as evidenced by the fact that they chose not to address safety issues in hospital facilities associated with non-acute care.

March and Olsen (1976), in their insightful analysis of organizational decision making, formulated what they called the Garbage Can Model of organizational decision making. In part, the model holds that problems and solutions exist in the same space and at the same time as independent streams. That is, many solutions do not come directly from an analysis of an extant problem, but, instead, they exist in the "ether." They float about in search of problems to which they might become attached. Seismic safety has long been attached to solutions having to do with seismically-resistant buildings. It is only natural that those concerned with treating those people injured in earthquakes would attach themselves almost automatically to a set of solutions requiring buildings that are more resistant to seismic motion, even though, for others, a number of other possibilities for treating the injured may come quickly to mind.

The record and our interviews with people who participated in framing the policy that became SB 1953 made it clear to us that they cared very much about ensuring the delivery of healthcare services to victims of a damaging earthquake. Their approach to the problem was to focus on ensuring the seismic resistance of facilities housing acute care hospital activities. They might have examined alternative ways to provide healthcare services to the injured in the event hospitals were damaged or considered the challenge of getting the injured to acute care hospitals through the earthquake damage and debris, but they did not. If they were concerned with not only treatment of the injured, but the well-being of existing patients, why, then, did they limit their focus to acute care facilities? We believe they framed the problem the way they did because the professional orientation of most of the people who framed the problem was building seismically safe structures. That, coupled with a failure to incorporate an understanding that many, if not most, hospitals are built episodically over time with additions to older buildings, helped lead to a policy that was particularly difficult to implement. The problem was defined primarily by structural engineers and seismologist who are, by their mindset, generally predisposed to think in terms of stronger structures as the solution to seismic safety.

A more reasoned approach to framing the problem might have been possible. Those persons concerned about seismic safety and the post-event functionality of hospitals might have formed a group comprising seismic safety advocates, hospital administrators, health care providers, and emergency managers to frame the problem and to devise an array of potential solutions that came closer to meeting the needs of those various parties that would, of necessity, be a party to any proposed solution. In all of our work on hazard mitigation for more than 25 years, we have yet to see that happen. More often than not, the advocates of some policy to enhance safety against an extreme event seem to assume that they know in advance, without having talked with them, that other stakeholders will take positions to oppose the advocates at every turn. Thus, the advocates seem to conclude that the only way to achieve their ends is to use everything at their disposal to overpower or to preempt other stakeholders so the policy they will be enacted as they want it, while making as few compromises as possible. Power politics are divisive. When there is significant interest and value overlap among various stakeholder parties as to ends and means, one might hope for collaboration.

It has been said that policy is made by those who have nothing better to do. That is not a slur on policy makers: it is simply recognition that those who are most politically actively involved in a particular issue are those for whom it has a very high priority. The term "zealot" refers to an activist with a single cause: one who pursues that cause with single-minded purpose. The word carries with it the connotation of a person whose mind is made up and with whom one cannot reason as she or he pursues the cause with unrelenting gusto. Zealots tend to see things primarily from a single perspective and tend to have strong beliefs about the righteousness of their cause. They often view those who do not agree with how they have framed the problem as not only wrong, but actually supporting malevolent positions. There is little doubt that a few of those who framed the policies embodied in SB 1953 were zealots: one State of California official, referring to the owners of hospitals not in compliance with the Alfred E. Alquist Hospital Facility Seismic Safety Act of 1973 told us "They've had 30 years to fix this problem and, by God, they're going to do it now."

We are not naïve. We understand that objective problem and policy analysis is a rarity, particularly in societies, like the United States, with deep and persistent ideological schisms. It is clear that many of those in policy making positions have little interest in gaining a deeper understanding of the complexities interwoven in policy issues. It seems, too, that ideology often has more to do with defining problems and solutions than to demonstrated facts. Policy, it is said, tastes like a stew made of elephant and rabbit, with the elephant being emotional and ideological reaction and the rabbit being careful, thoughtful analysis. It would take a lot more rabbits than we currently put into the stew to alter the dominant elephant taste.

12.2.3 Factors Affecting Problem Framing

12.2.3.1 Government Structure: Silos Within Silos, Spheres of Mutual Non Intervention, and Institutionalized Access

How we've organized our governments contributes considerably to how problems are framed and solutions are selected. A central structural problem is that government executive agencies are usually organized in terms of delivering services by topical function. Operating within functional silos, they are hard-pressed to address the many significant problems that cut across agency interests and functional responsibilities. The legislative branch is often organized on essentially the same basis, except with a greater emphasis on clientele base and interest groups. The chief executive is presumably in a position to examine problems and consider priorities based on their respective contributions to addressing the major problems, but we do not see that happening very often. On rare occasion, a chief executive will make a bold move and create a matrix-based organization to address problems that cut across functions and that may vary geographically; they usually work for a while and then, when the executive moves on or the energy required to keep the system from slipping back into its old and more comfortable modes dissipates, and the agencies, bureaus, and offices quickly reorganize back into the traditional pattern.[2]

To make matters worse, larger agencies within the bureaucracies are further organized by subtopic. Illustratively, most environmental protection agencies regulate air and water discharges through separate organizational entities even though the two vehicles for transporting pollutants are almost inextricably linked. Illustratively, airborne deposition of pollutants is a major factor in water pollution by mercury, polychlorinated biphenyls (PCBs), and other volatile toxins. A discharger can sometimes choose which vehicle by which to discharge the regulated material based on whether air or water regulations are tighter. It would, of course, make sense to regulate these matters by both the medium by which they are discharged into the environment and by geographic location, but that rarely, if ever, happens.

The silo-based structures that dominate both the executive and legislative branches of our local, state and federal governments make it extremely difficult to frame problems and devise policies that reflect the complexity of problems we face: the structure virtually ensures that problems will be framed sub-optimally, that too much will be spent on some narrowly construed problem and not enough on another problem that might be the focus of another organization and that could also be addressed at the same time.

The functional Balkanization of individual governments contributes to the political phenomenon known as spheres of mutual non intervention. The term is usually used in connection with legislative bodies; it refers to the practice in which various individuals or committees are given deference by the rest of the body when they propose courses of action having to do with their specific set of interests and knowledge. In the case of SB 1953, Senator Alfred Alquist experienced that kind of deference when it came to earthquake legislation. He championed most of the State's seismic safety legislation and was viewed as *the* authority within the legislature. He, of course, did not experience that level of deference in other topical matters where other legislators enjoyed that level of deference.

This brings us to another phenomenon that contributes to framing problems and selecting solutions that are clearly (to outside observers) sub-optimal. This is the phenomenon of institutionalized access. Institutionalized access exists when a

---

[2]Wayne Thompson, City Manager of Oakland, California, headed the Ford Foundation's first Gray Area Project in 1962. Thompson employed a matrix over the City's traditional organization so that municipal agencies would collectively focus on specific problems in specific neighborhoods. See the *American Journal of Public Health*, November, 1967. Vol. 57. No. 11, page 2,055. George Maier, Secretary of the Wisconsin Department of Natural Resources was able, for a brief time, to organize that agency by watersheds within central functional specialties to assist the heads of watersheds deal with cross-cutting problems. See D. J. Alesch, *New Strategies for Environmental Problems in Wisconsin: Breaking Out of the Box*. Thiensville, WI: Wisconsin Policy Research Institute, February 1997.

specific interest has automatic and preferred access to specific government decision making bodies relative to an area of interest. In the matter of earthquake policy, the California State Seismic Safety Commission has institutionalized access to State decision makers on matters of earthquake policy. The Commission "investigates earthquakes, researches earthquake-related issues and reports, and recommends to the Governor and Legislature policies and programs needed to reduce earthquake risk" (State Seismic Safety Commission 2011). The Commission is governed by 20 commissioners who are chosen for their expertise and experience in various aspects of earthquakes and earthquake safety. Fifteen members are appointed by the Governor and confirmed by the Senate, one member is appointed by the Senate Rules Committee, and one member is appointed by the Speaker of the Assembly. There are three *ex officio* members: one each from the State's Building Standards Commission, the State Architect's office, and the State's Emergency Management Agency.

The Seismic Safety Commission advocates policies to enhance seismic safety. It is not charged with addressing the broader problems of healthcare and hospital service in California, so it is only natural that it limited its framing of the old hospital problem to ensuring the seismic resistance of hospital structures.

Even though it has been a very long time since anyone has died in a California earthquake in a hospital, even though many die in those hospitals from other preventable reasons, one should not expect the State Seismic Safety Commission to speak out for addressing other healthcare problems before addressing seismic safety in hospitals. This is not a criticism of the agency; it was doing its job in laying the groundwork for SB 1953. The problem is one of government structure and the fact that the job of setting priorities among competing interests and problems apparently belongs to someone else. Unfortunately, in most places in this country, no one seems to know who that is.

12.2.3.2 Causal Models and Chance Events

Pressman and Wildavsky (1973) argue that poorly designed programs – those with internal inconsistencies or that put impossible or silly requirements on the target population – are unlikely to work. Policies must be based on a valid causal model if they are to work. Sabatier and Mazmanian (1979) agree and state the proposition succinctly: "For a policy to be implemented effectively, the … (policy must be) based on a sound theory relating changes in target group behavior to the achievement of the desired end-state" (Sabatier and Mazmanian 1979).

A causal model is an abstraction that employs cause and effect logic to describe the relationships between independent and dependent variables. Humans employ causal models, both consciously and subconsciously, when they say or think "If I do *this*, then *that* will follow." The logic underlying policies is typically based on a belief in "if x, then y." The belief may be based on ideological or religious beliefs, on hope, or on scientific evidence: it usually does not matter which in the eyes of the advocate. The basic model on which SB 1953 is based is this: If we enact a law requiring owners of acute care hospital to retrofit, replace, or take from service old, unsafe hospitals and, if we threaten serious consequences for not complying, then hospital owners will comply and they will comply in accord with the timeline we have set forth.

Unfortunately two major problems exist with respect to causal models. The first is that they (usually) work really well in laboratories under controlled conditions. They are a lot less reliable when applied to large scale socio-economic and behavioral systems. The second reason is that we get them wrong too many times. We reason from past events and simplifying assumptions. To compound the problem, we assume that our causal models are based on conditions of certainty. That is, because we created the model carefully, we believe that is will work as planned: if we do this thing, that thing will occur with no chance of error or adverse consequences. Clearly, that is naïve, but we humans still have a tendency to do it.

The more appropriate approach is to understand from the start that we live in a world where outcomes are rarely certain. Classical decision theory provides normative guides to decision making under three and only three formally defined conditions: certainty, risk, and uncertainty. *Certainty* is defined as a condition in which we know exactly what will happen as a consequence of a choice. There is no room for a chance event or a chance outcome. Personally, we have never encountered such a situation, but were we to, decision making would be easy. *Risk* is defined as a situation in which we know all the possible outcomes stemming from an action, and the probability distribution of each occurring. *Uncertainty* is defined as a condition in which we know all the possible outcomes from an action but not the probability distribution of each of them occurring. Except in trivial, mechanical, or chemical matters, this condition exists only rarely.

In the matter of public policy decision making, we do not believe that any of those three conditions can exist. We do not believe that one can list all the possible outcomes of an action. Decision-event trees that are constructed following the logic of decision making under conditions of uncertainty are useful as guides to thinking, but, often, the real, concrete situation about which one proposes to make a choice about action is simply too fraught with uncertainty to use the model alone. That is why we think in terms of *partial information* and *ignorance* as the primary conditions under which policy is made, rather than any of the classical constructs. Partial information is a condition in which the decision maker may know some of the outcomes that might occur if a policy or program is promulgated, but not all of them. Decision making under conditions of ignorance is much like "If I do x, then I have no idea what will happen." Unfortunately, decision makers working under conditions of partial information or ignorance too often imagine themselves as working under conditions of certainty.

12.2.3.3 Ideology and Politics

Understanding how problems are formulated becomes more complex when we add a consideration of varying ideological beliefs and politics to the mix. Ideological differences between people and groups affect how problems are framed and the perceived validity of various causal models. For example, Keynesians believe that it is appropriate for government to increase spending in times of recession or depression to stimulate the economy. Those who trust Friedrich Hayek believe that governments should decrease expenditures to stimulate the economy. It might be said that they, along with Tea Party members, believe governments should reduce expenditures under any conditions. Ideology shapes what one perceives and reality for humans is based on perceptions.

Politics are not always shaped by ideology, but in a jurisdiction where ideological beliefs run strong and counter to one another, the middle ground, which may tend toward pragmatism, often shrinks in proportion to the extreme positions. That makes problem framing less a matter of thoughtful analysis than a matter of who can shout the loudest or who can garner the most votes at any given time.

We do not believe that ideology had much of a role in shaping SB 1953 or in the California's legislature's decision not to provide either money or incentives to help public and private hospitals respond to the legislative mandates. It seems to us that the State government was simply unwilling to increase taxes or to transfer some of its existing resources from other activities to fund the effort; the competition for dollars, the reluctance to increase taxes, and the desire not to alienate other interests seems sufficient to explain the behavior.

12.3 The Policy Itself and the Program Design as Obstacles

How a policy is framed and how the program intended to implement it is designed makes a significant difference in the likelihood that the program and the underlying policy will be implemented successfully. Anyone can design a program, but a well-designed program is rare and a thing of beauty – at least for those of us who care about such things. We find that several considerations are critical in policy and program design.

12.3.1 Matching the Policy and the Program to the Problem

Mazmanian and Sabatier (1989) remind us that some public problems are simply much easier to deal with than others. Certainly, this is the case with old hospital facilities that do not comply with current seismic standards. Sometimes, the charter of the agency involved with the policy and program do not match the breadth and complexity of the problem. Consequently, the agency and its advocates focus on the aspect of the problem for which they do have domain. When that happens, policies and programs may not match the basic problem. When one steps back to try to understand in a broader context why hospital owners own buildings that do not meet current seismic standards, it is probably not because they have little concern for the safety of patients and staff. Stepping back, one might also see that the hospital facilities were deficient in some other areas: it appears that many of the pre-1973 hospital facilities classified as seismically unsafe were also inefficient and outmoded in terms of today's medical practices and labor costs and should have been replaced simply to enhance efficiency. All the evidence, though, demonstrates that most hospital owners simply did not have sufficient financial resources to either retrofit or replace their facilities. Finally, stepping back from the initial focus would have made it clear that many of the buildings not meeting standards were located in rural or poverty stricken areas and that obtaining adequate healthcare was beyond the financial capability of many Californians.

Taken altogether, the healthcare problem may actually have been intractable. It might still be. When problems are intractable, it makes sense to write legislation that expresses goals and means for accomplishing those goals. It doesn't make sense to include a lockstep set of deadlines when intervening in an incredibly complex and dynamic system, especially when the workings of that system are poorly understood and there are likely to be unpredictable consequences of the intervention. When systemic relationships within a complex set of phenomena are not well understood or when there is no agreement about how to approach a complex, multidimensional problem, then almost any policy has a significant chance of not achieving the desired outcomes and of having serious adverse side effects. The more intractable a problem toward which a policy is directed is perceived, the less likely it is that implementation will be successful. Intractability can result because we are ignorant about a phenomenon that concerns us, because the target population is large and diverse, or because the challenge of changing behavior in a large segment of a large, diverse target population is overwhelming.

Clearly, both continued ignorance or somewhat improved scientific or technical understanding can be major obstacles in the policy formulation process. The failed steel welds phenomenon is a good example. Sometimes, it takes considerable time before any level of agreement can be reached concerning whether a problem exists at all. Some hold, for example, that global warming is well underway and has dire consequences. Others argue that there is inadequate evidence of global warming. Still others argue that global warming could trigger a new ice age. Unfortunately, we are sometimes unable to agree that a problem exists until it is too late to do anything about it.

The drive for performance-based seismic design standards provides an illustration that is informative, but not as complex as the old hospital problem. Performance-based seismic design standards have been a focus of attention among those in California concerned with seismic safety for a decade or more: performance-based design makes lots of sense. The approach embraces the notion that performance specifications are superior to specifications-based standards to the extent that they provide an incentive for innovation in design, materials, and construction. Moreover, buildings intended for different uses should probably be built to different standards. One set of proposals, however, suggested that in California, performance requirements might decline in some proportion to the distance between the site and known faults. That idea became less compelling as it became clear that the Northridge earthquake along with some other damaging earthquakes in California took place on previously unknown faults.

New knowledge and new perceptions often render policy recommendations or existing policies irrelevant – ideas that made a lot of sense at the time they were proposed or enacted. Sabatier and Mazmanian (1979) believe that shifting conditions can undermine implementation even after a policy is enacted, because the shifts may lead to new public policies that conflict with existing policies.

12.3.2 Policy Making Is Inherently Political

For those who despair of politics, wishing instead that hazard mitigation were simply given to technical experts, it is important to remember that mitigation almost always requires allocating and reallocating resources; it is inherently political. Since a significant portion of politics involves manipulating content and symbols for purposes of gaining political support, one should not be surprised when policy is enacted that few policy makers actually expect to be implemented or when policy outputs do not resemble the result you might expect, given the inputs you thought you saw. Long ago, in another case study, we concluded that "Hazard mitigation is not a technical exercise; it is inherently and often intensely political because mitigation usually involves placing cost burdens on some stakeholders, and may involve a redistribution of resources. Hazard mitigators must, therefore, develop political as well as technical solutions" (Alesch and Petak 1986, p. 227). Hazard mitigators, in our experience, are frequently willing to require other people to spend more of their money on hazard mitigation than they want to or may be able to afford, given other priorities. On the other hand, most people seem to discount low probability/high consequence events heavily, have faulty perceptions about the probabilities of extreme events and resultant consequences, and often expect others to bear their losses when the event occurs. Because values and perception are so different among stakeholders, it is difficult, if not impossible to reach consensus about appropriate mitigation policy interventions.

It didn't take 50 years for Los Angeles to pass a unreinforced masonry building retrofit ordinance because the structural engineering problems were so difficult to address. It took that long because hazard mitigators continued to offer technical solutions to a problem that inherently involved a redistribution of costs, income, and wealth. The ordinance passed only when the redistribution problems were addressed in a way that a critical mass of support could be assembled and held together until after the vote. Lester Thurow (1980) makes the point in his *Zero-Sum Society* that we have created a society with so much access to public policy makers that almost anybody can stop anything. And, "anybody" is often willing to very work hard to stop a policy that threatens his or her financial well-being.

Because stakeholders in hazard mitigation politics have dramatically different perceptions of the situation and hold different perceptions of risks and outcomes, achieving sufficient political agreement on a mitigation policy requires that trade-offs be made among the extent of the hazard reduction, the total costs of mitigation, who pays for various mitigation costs, the level of safety to be achieved, and the timetable for accomplishment. If, for some reason, those trade-offs are not made during policy and program design, they are likely, as they did in the case of SB 1953, after the legislation is enacted and program regulations are promulgated; i.e., during implementation.

12.3.3 The Agency Role in Policy Design

Policymaking is not entirely the domain of elected officials. Obviously, interested parties bring candidates for policy to the attention of legislators and chief executives, but so do government agencies. Executive agencies charged with policy implementation usually design the programs that operationalize the policy. Agencies are typically required to draft rules and then to seek comments from those who have an interest in those rules or to hold public hearings to garner input. Parties with a stake in the outcome testify and otherwise pressure the agency to have the regulations reflect their interests. In the end, the agency decides what the rules will be. Sometimes, but not always, those rules must be ratified by another body. Once adopted, the administrative regulations have the force of law and, thus, become public policy.

Within the broad statements of a policy, room often exists for agencies to choose from a broad array of program designs. The SB 1953 policy was intended, from the start, as a regulatory program. The 3 years during which OSHPD worked to develop the rules resulted in a program design that resulted in a very large proportion of the acute care hospital facilities in California in need of virtually immediate action to reduce seismic risk. One basis for program designs is a careful analysis of the likely outcomes and consequences of one approach over another. Another approach is to devise the program in terms of what appears to be politically possible. The former approach is preferred by many, but the latter approach often dictates what happens, particularly in contentious circumstances. Still, it remains a mystery to us why the SB 1953 program regulations were devised so that so many hospital facilities would require immediate action at such great cost, particularly during a period in which all the evidence indicated that such a large proportion of hospitals was in dire financial straits and there were no resources at the State level to provide any financial support or incentives and few resources within the hospital industry with which to carry out the mandated improvements

We believe that the complexity of the program required to implement a given policy affects the probability of successful implementation. That does not mean we argue for simplicity for the sake of simplicity, nor does it mean that we believe any simple program has a better chance of being successful than any complicated program. It means this: programs should never be more complex than they have to be or involve more actors than are absolutely needed. Sociotechnical systems analysts refer to designing things to "minimal critical specifications." The criteria for classifying hospitals as unsafe in earthquakes may have been, in retrospect, over-specified. Given the large number of hospital facilities so classified, the timetable for implementation was probably too demanding. OSHPD's response to the challenge was to introduce the

HAZUS model, which, had it been available at the time, would have been far superior to the variables employed in the first classification go-round. On the other hand, one might argue that the high standards and the tight timetable brought an important issue to the fore and stimulated investment in new hospitals. It might even have been anticipated by advocates that adjustments might be made in the timetable to ease the burden on those hospitals in particularly difficult circumstances.

12.3.4 The Choice of Instrumentality: How to Achieve the Desired Ends

Regulatory policies, though often employed to effect policy objectives, are only one of many ways to accomplish public policy objectives. Petak and Atkisson (1982, p. 61) list other "types of hazard-related public policies" from which policy makers might choose an appropriate means for achieving one or more outcomes in a targeted system. The list includes, among others, attention-focusing policies, technology development policies, investment policies, and direct actions in which government is authorized to implement a policy, "such as physical construction or removal of structures."

One of the most important characteristics of program design is that policy makers have a tendency to reach for mechanisms and approaches they've used before when designing programs. SB 1953 is clearly a regulatory policy. It directs private organizations (not-for-profit and investor-owned organizations) as well as other public jurisdictions within the State to retrofit, replace, or take from use acute care hospital facilities that do not meet specified standards. Given the tumult in the healthcare industry at the time and the large proportion of hospitals, might not other implementation strategies have been considered?

The State government obviously has the right and the power to order acute care hospital owners to comply with the law or face loss of their respective licenses. This is, in its rawest form, a pricing policy. The State intended to raise the costs of noncompliance to a level that no hospital owner would be willing to pay. Since a number of hospitals simply went out of business, the price was apparently either not high enough to compel the desired behavior or too high for some players to pay.

Raising the cost of noncompliance is not the only way to use pricing to achieve public policy objectives. The State could have lowered the costs of complying while simultaneously raising the costs for not complying. That is, the State could choose to provide incentives for doing what it deemed to be "the right thing" and, at the same time, raise the costs of not doing it. The policy selected by the State was not "the carrot or the stick" but only "the stick." The State chose an approach that is sometimes called "bureaucratic bludgeoning."

The cost of complying was clearly the primary obstacle to hospitals for not complying and for struggling to find ways of delaying the inevitable need to comply with the law. The State could have, without allocating hard dollars to hospitals, found ways to reduce the costs of complying. For investor-owned hospitals, the

State might have proposed accelerated depreciation or investment tax credits. It could have provided a revolving loan fund. It might have chosen to enter into contracts with individual hospitals to have those hospitals stage their seismic safety enhancements through some timetable rather than stipulating a "one size fits all" timetable. The State might have examined the array of hospitals within various service areas and selected one or two as priority facilities to serve in the event of a damaging earthquake while, at the same time, working with the other hospitals to achieve the objective of seismic safety and continued functionality.

There exists a myriad of ways for government to achieve its policy objectives without imposing regulations perceived by the targeted organizations as onerous or as virtually impossible to meet given their other legitimate obligations. Too often, it seems government agencies reach for the regulatory tool. Perhaps that is because they can or because they find it easier than devising other means that would work with fewer adverse side effects.

12.3.5 Path Dependency and Ignoring History

The solution to the "old hospitals without adequate seismic resistance" problem was essentially built into Steinbrugge's 1971 statement of the problem. From his perspective and those of his followers, the only solution considered was stronger buildings. As you may recall from an earlier reference, his statement was:

> Surely public interest is much better served if hospital structures are designed with sufficient damage control features so as to remain functional after an event. This means not only placing severe limits on permissible structural damage, but also severe limits on permissible elevator damage, telephone and other communications damage, standby power damage and the like (Steinbrugge et al. 1971, p. 56).

The solution obviously meant creating new standards for new hospital facilities and that was accomplished in 1973 and again in 1983. SB 1953 extended the solution to pre-existing facilities.

At both the state and local levels, statutes and ordinances requiring that buildings built before one or another standard was added to the building code have always experienced hard times in California. SB 1953 was patterned after the Field Act. The Field Act has been under attack by various interests since it was enacted more than 75 years ago. Until recently, some unreinforced masonry buildings that were to be replaced as a consequence of the Act still remained in service as school buildings. The most recent attacks on the Field Act have been the attempt by California's community colleges to be exempted from the law so they could cuts costs.

A second example also has to do with retrofitting, replacing, or removing unreinforced masonry buildings from service. This example stems from municipal ordinances rather than state statutes. Building officials in the City of Long Beach, California, epicenter of the 1933 Long Beach Earthquake, tried desperately to get the city council to enact ordinances to retrofit or remove unreinforced masonry buildings and to make those ordinances stick. Time after time, ordinances were passed and then watered down or rescinded until one finally stuck in the 1970s. The City of Los Angeles tried to enact unreinforced masonry building retrofit laws as well. It took Los Angeles more than 50 years, 10 years longer than Long Beach, to enact an ordinance that stuck. And, it took California years after that to adopt a model ordinance for other municipalities and that model required minimal improvements. One important reason for the troubled history of unreinforced masonry (URM) ordinances was that most of those with a stake in the outcome of the proposed policies had divergent perceptions of the problem. Building officials, looking at unreinforced masonry buildings, saw a public safety problem. Owners of the unreinforced masonry buildings saw them as a source of income and URM retrofit proposals as a serious threat to their income flow and the value of their asset. Occupants valued the buildings as a generally low cost place to live or do business and saw the policy proposals leading to an almost certain increase in rent or as a threat to continued occupancy.

The problems associated with enacting building retrofit legislation have not gone unnoticed by social scientists. Two of the authors of this work explained in a 1985 book that the Long Beach and Los Angeles retrofit ordinances required political solutions as much as technical solutions (Alesch and Petak 1986). It is difficult to understand why, if something has regularly not worked well in the past, the advocates of SB 1953 would think it would work well this time. Albert Einstein described the futility of doing the same thing over and over again and expecting different results.

Why, then, would seismic safety advocates recommend employing essentially the same approach to addressing the old building problem that has not worked in the past? Three possibilities are plausible. First, they might not have really understood the problems encountered by the Field Act and the unreinforced masonry building ordinances. Second, they might not have seen any other plausible solution to the problem. The third, and in our minds, the most likely is that they were caught up in dual traps of forgetting history and path dependency.

Path dependency refers to following a course of action that already exists as a paradigm or that has already been initiated and has some momentum. Path dependency occurs because it is often easier to continue along a set path than to create an entirely new one. For us, it seems clear that the initial problem statement phrased by Karl Steinbrugge a quarter century ago created a path-dependent starting point for the problem definition embodied in SB 1953. In any case, what he wrote in 1971 had significant staying power.

12.3.6 A Lack of Congruence Between the Policy and the Prerequisites to Action for the Targeted Organizations

In an earlier chapter, we identified what we believe to be prerequisites to organizational action. SB 1953 was formulated and enacted apparently without considering that, for a very large majority of acute care hospitals in the State, the requirements of the program were incongruent with the prerequisites to action for those targeted organizations. Specifically, as much as 85% of the acute care hospitals did not have adequate resources to undertake either structural retrofit or replacement. Therefore, it was extremely unlikely that implementation would proceed as anticipated by program administrators. Only those few hospital owners with positive margins, adequate cash flow, and sufficient access to the capital required to retrofit or replace would be able to comply according to the deadlines.

If public regulatory policy is to be implemented without ruinous consequences, it must be congruous with the legitimate needs and basic prerequisites to action for those organizations expected to *actually* implement the policy.

Many of those who championed a policy like SB 1953 called for the State to provide financial assistance and incentives for hospitals to comply, but the State chose not to provide either financial assistance or incentives for hospital owners. Most acute care hospital owners in the State were in serious financial trouble just when they were supposed to comply with the statute; most saw the problem of how to comply as intractable. We have heard a very small number of SB 1953 advocates say that they did not believe the hospital owners when they said they did not have sufficient resources to comply. In any event, the fact that many hospitals were in dire financial conditions and could not have complied with the 2008 deadline was a critical factor in the implementation problems that became apparent.

12.3.7 Establishing Unrealistic Demands

If public policies are to be implemented on a timely basis, it is imperative that they provide sufficient time for targeted organizations to comply. SB 1953 did not. The program regulations established a timeline that was essentially impossible to meet even under the best of circumstances.

The law was enacted in September 21, 1994, but the program regulations were not issued until March 18, 1998. The law and the administrative code called for 1,027 hospital buildings that were classified as SPC-1 on January 1, 2001 to be made safe, replaced, or removed from service in just 7 years, by January 1, 2008. Seven years is close to the minimum time required from project initiation to final project completions for complex facilities. If one assumes 1 year for creating an approximation of the final project and to arrange financing, which we have found in our experience to be almost a minimum, then only 6 years remain for OSHPD to review and approve the plans, to acquire or clear land, and to complete detailed design, conduct value engineering, complete construction, complete equipping and furnishing, conduct training, and to work through final punch lists and complete inspections. Had there been fewer than 100 hospital buildings that had to be repaired or replaced, it might have been done. With more than 1,000 buildings facing the same task set, we doubt that there were sufficient numbers of structural engineers and architects capable and experienced in hospital design and sufficient numbers of contractors to complete the job. This is especially the case when each of the facilities would be seeking financing at the same time, finding designers at the same time, seeking OSHPD approval at the same time, relocating patients and structures at the same time, and then building at the same time.

Unless those who wrote the legislation meant to create a crisis requiring hospital owners to initiate action with the expectation of making adjustments as to when compliance was really expected for various hospitals, the policy was unworkable from the start. No one appears to have thought through the *systemic* complexity of retrofitting or rebuilding 1,000 plus hospital buildings in a short time frame. On the simplest level of analysis, how many employees would OSHPD have needed in the year when it was most involved in plan checking, etc. only to have many of those same employees idle in subsequent years when the demands for their services would have diminished significantly? Even from a work planning perspective, the timeline was unrealistic.

12.4 In Summary: Barriers to Effective Implementation and Implications for Policy Design

12.4.1 Barriers

The processes involved in public intervention in problematic situations encompass problem articulation and formulation, interest aggregation, policy formation, policy enactment, implementation and administration, and, sometimes, policy adaptation. These processes are structured in terms of how government is organized and how roles are assigned to various components of the government or taken on by those components. The processes are activated by individuals, groups, and organizations with interests in procedural and substantive issues. The activated processes take place in any number of locations, across agency lines, across levels of government, and between governments at the same level.

From our perspective, the implementation segment of the larger policymaking and implementation process is anything but linear and predictable or even iterative. Instead, it is dynamic and interactive. We sometimes describe it as stochastic and nondeterministic because, so often, it involves large numbers of disparate actors with disparate concerns, aspirations, and strategies. While one can sketch in the broad outlines of the implementation process, it is much more problematic to draw inferences about how the process will unfold in any individual case. In our experience, implementation activities lead to adaptive behaviors on the part of participants. Policymaking is inherently political. To the extent that implementers are involved in shaping or altering policy during the design period or as programs are administered, they, too, are engaged in political activities.

Taken together, the implementation process seems to us to resemble a large, loosely constructed, self-organizing cluster of interests, actors, legalities, organizations, and issues. It appears to be almost amorphous, forming around issues and then, not disassociating but, rather, refocusing on other, related issues, often with changes in the membership. Some elements in the process are persistent and remain active over an extended time period in a set of related issues. Other elements coalesce around specific issues and then move into the background where they become latent interests and interest groups, ready to manifest themselves and join in again at such time as their interests are sufficiently threatened.

Several primary forces within the implementation process have a considerable affect on the extent to which the aims stated in a public policy actually result in the desired outcomes. First among these is the design of the policy itself and the program intended to accomplish the objectives stated in the policy. To what extent does the policy embody a problem statement that makes sense and an innate causal model that, in the words of Sabatier and Mazmanian (1979) is "based on a sound theory relating changes in target group behavior to the achievement of the desired end-state?" Another primary force is the extent to which both the policy and the program designed to bring about the desired outcomes is compatible with the prerequisites to action for the targeted organizations. If the policy or program is incongruent with those prerequisites, successful implementation is unlikely. A third primary force in implementation is the extent to which the behaviors, policies, and actions of the administering agency or agencies are compatible with and supportive of the substantive intent of the policy. If an agency at one level of government is dependent on agencies within that level of government or in other levels of government to actually take the desired actions or to cause others to take those actions, then the integrity of that network is critically important to successful implementation.

12.4.2 Implications for Policy Design

The implications of our findings about the barriers to public policy implementation for policy and program design are fairly straightforward. They begin with how the problem is framed. We know that some elected officials propose legislation based on bad science, ignorance, and political opportunism. Nonetheless, metaphorically walking around the dark crystal and peering into the various cloudy lenses can help to frame the problem in such a way that it makes sense to those who are seriously seeking some acceptable solution.

We have concluded that the likelihood of successful implementation depends on the extent to which all those involved in the implementation network have shared perceptions of existing conditions, have compatible perceptions of desirable end-states, and generally agree on the appropriate means for achieving the desired end-state. The likelihood of complete concurrence is, of course, extraordinarily unlikely. Organizations have a tendency to suboptimize in terms of the breadth of their responsibility. Building departments can define problems in terms of their responsibilities without paying a great deal of attention to other concerns in the city. That is, they can think in terms of removing buildings with relatively low seismic resistance from the housing stock without giving too much thought to the possible displacement of lower income households. City planners cannot. The city council cannot. Building owners can similarly suboptimize to focus the problem definition on their building and their bank accounts.

Then, if the policy is based on a reasonably reliable causal model and if it is congruent with the prerequisites to action of the organizations expected to take the action needed to bring about the desired outcomes, and if the policy provides the administrative agency with appropriate tools, we might have reason to hope for successful implementation.

Enacting policy and assigning responsibility does not take the policy maker off the hook; unanticipated consequences abound, so it is necessary to monitor the consequences of the policy. Any shortcomings in the policy or adverse consequences require timely, sensible adaptation to the circumstances. Legislating without monitoring consequences and fixing inequities is irresponsible. Nonetheless, it happens.

Finally, the executive and the legislators must ensure that the administering agency has the resources it needs to conduct its operations effectively and on a timely basis. Cutting back on staffing, imposing needlessly burdensome administrative rules, and being niggardly in terms of financial resources can result in serious and mounting administrative obstacles.

References

Ackoff R (1974) Redesigning the future. Wiley, New York

Alesch D, Petak W (1986) The politics and economics of earthquake hazard mitigation: unreinforced masonry buildings in Southern California. Institute of Behavioral Science, University of Colorado, Boulder

Arrow K (1951) Social choice and individual values. Wiley, New York

Crowley CF, Nalder E (2009) Dead by mistake: within health care hides massive, avoidable death. Hearst newspapers, August 10. http://www.chron.com/disp/story.mpl/deadbymistake/6555095.html

Lasswell HD (1976) Power and personality. W. W. Norton & Company, Inc., New York

March JG, Olsen JP (1976) Ambiguity and choice in organizations. Unversitetsforlaget, Bergen

Mazmanian DA, Sabatier PA (1989) Implementation and public policy: with a new postscript. University Press of America

Petak WJ, Atkisson AA (1982) Natural hazard risk assessment and public policy: anticipating the unexpected. Springer, New York, Lanham, MD

Pressman JL, Wildavsky A (1973) Implementation. University of California Press, Berkeley

Sabatier P, Mazmanian D (1979) The conditions of effective implementation; a guide to accomplishing policy objectives. Policy Anal 5:481–504

State Seismic Safety Commission (2011). Official California Seismic Safety Commission website home page. http://www.seismic.ca.gov/

Steinbrugge KE, Schader BH, Weers C (1971) San Fernando earthquake, February 9,1971. Pacific Fire Rating Bureau, San Francisco, August 10

Thurow LC (1980) The zero-sum society: distribution and the possibilities for economic change. Basic Books, New York

Chapter 13
Dynamic Contexts and Public Policy Implementation

13.1 Causal Textures, Butterflies, and Black Swans

Chapter 12 focused on the implementation process itself and the obstacles to implementation that can and often do arise in that process. This chapter focuses on another set of variables that often affect the extent to which policy is or can be implemented effectively. That set of variables has to do with the dynamics of the context within which those engaged in the various parts of implementation find themselves.

Obviously, implementation does not occur in a vacuum. Non-governmental organizations expected to comply with new regulations typically find themselves responding not only to the new regulation, but to other phenomena emerging from other sources and particularly salient to their primary activities. In a dynamic context, events can occur and conditions can arise that quickly alter the focus of an organization and its ability to deal with items on last week's agenda. Consequently, it is foolish to assume that, once put into effect, a program can continue in place without being altered and still have the desired outcomes. When policies and programs are not flexible and when governments are unable to adopt policy changes quickly to adapt to significant changes in context, continued attempts to stay the course inevitably lead to unanticipated and undesirable outcomes.

Many of the variables within the policy making and implementation process can, at least to some extent, be controlled. At the very least, participants in the process may be able to exert some influence over how the process plays out. A dynamic context, though, develops largely apart and separate from the policy making and implementation process. This is not to say that there might not be some interaction between the process and the context; we're inclined to believe in the existence of interacting and interdependent sets of events and conditions. We do mean to say that those involved in the policymaking and implementation process are often conscious of the interplay and processes outside their milieu, but sometimes not quite understanding the implications for them. We have concluded that the outcomes of SB 1953, at least through 2010, are as much a function of a dynamic external environment

D.J. Alesch et al., *Natural Hazard Mitigation Policy: Implementation, Organizational Choice, and Contextual Dynamics*, Environmental Hazards, DOI 10.1007/978-94-007-2235-4_13, © Springer Science+Business Media B.V. 2012

as they are of the way the problem was defined, the law written, and the regulations drafted and adopted.

The outcomes of any intervention in a large complex system are largely unpredictable. There are almost always unanticipated consequences; things rarely work out as expected. To the extent that policy makers and program designers do not internalize those realities, program implementation suffers. Policy making and program implementation obviously take place within a context and that context affects programmatic success. Sabatier (1986) concludes that changes in socioeconomic conditions sometimes undermine the causal theory or political support for specific policies. Calista (1994) adds public opinion and interpretive institutions, such as courts, to the policy environment. It makes sense. We believe, for example, that the contexts of the Great Depression and World War II delayed serious concern of unreinforced masonry buildings in southern California.

We subscribe to the notion that the consequences of actions taken are subject to large doses of chance and more often than not result in unanticipated outcomes. Actions are taken, consequences result, and sequences of successive outcomes cascade outward. Sometimes the chain of consequences attenuates; other times it does not. When one drops a rock of any significant size into a puddle of water, one cannot anticipate all the possible ripples. The unpredictability of consequences varies with the characteristics of the environment within which policies and programs are implemented; they can range from somewhat predictable to highly unpredictable. The "texture" of the environment affects how the targeted system responds to the intervention in its workings or its environment.

As mentioned earlier, half a century ago, Emery and Trist (1965) wrote an extremely insightful article entitled *The Causal Texture of Organizational Environments*. In the article, they define four kinds of causal textures within which an organization might exist at any given time. Their analysis can be extended beyond the environment of the individual firm to embrace decision making contexts more generally.

The first of Emery and Trist's causal textures is *placid-random*. Within the placid-random environment, relationships are generally stable and persistent. Shocks to the system are random and cannot be predicted reliably. Within that context, decision making is relatively simple and simple cause and effect models are generally sufficient; i.e., one can generally predict the consequences of taking an action, subject to an unexpected jolt from some randomly occurring event.

The second causal texture is called the *placid-clustered* texture. In this context, strategy and tactics are differentiated from one another. In the context of our discussion about public policy, the ability to predict the array of outcomes in a system from intervening in it is much less predictable. Relationships among elements in the system are more transient and less predictable. The third causal texture exhibits still more complexity and considerably more uncertainty about the consequences of action. It is called a *disturbed-reactive environment*. This is an environment within which the actions of one actor or element within the system result in largely unpredictable actions by other actors or elements. Often these actions are taken in an attempt to thwart those of the initiating party or parties. That is, when one takes action, others can be expected to take unexpected kinds of action so that the consequences of your action become increasingly less predictable.

The fourth causal texture is called the *turbulent field*. The turbulent field is a decision making context within which very little is predictable with reliability. Causal relationships are not durable, they change, and the consequences of action or inaction may be completely unanticipated.

This brief discussion does not do justice to the concepts outlined by Emery, Trist, and others, but it is sufficient to suggest why policies calling for significant action, once put in place, cannot be left alone without monitoring and adaptation as needed. If one assumes the policy environment to be stable and predictable both now and in the relevant future, one creates policies that are unlikely to have the desired consequences when the causal texture of the environment is not placid random. For the most part, placid-random environments are rare; more often, the environment is turbulent. Policy makers who create programs that they expect to be implemented over years, if not decades, and who fail to recognize the dynamic nature of the context within which they are operating, are likely setting those policies up for failure.

The fact that most contexts are dynamic means that they are changing continually or, at least, episodically. We do not expect public policy makers to be able to reliably predict how complex, dynamic systems will respond to the complex, dynamic environments in which they exist. And, most certainly, we do not expect public officials to be able to predict reliably how, when, and to what extent organizations will respond to policy mandates as their environments change as well.

Complex, dynamic systems comprising interrelated social, economic, and political components change continually. Usually, the changes are evolutionary as members of the system respond to cues from themselves or from others in the system and in its relevant environment. Sometimes, however, the changes are rapid and dramatic. This mix of evolutionary and revolutionary change is called punctuated equilibrium (Baumgartner and Jones 2009). These systems are generally self-organizing as the individual components make choices about what to do, where to do it, when to do it, and how to do it.[1] Future states of the system are typically extremely difficult to predict reliably, particularly when the system exists within a turbulent environment. The future conditions or states of various agents or sets of agents are similarly difficult to predict reliably.

The reasons for considerable uncertainty about the consequences of choice and action have to do with the superabundance of chance events in disturbed and turbulent environments – events over which we have little or no control as to their occurrence or outcomes. One formulation contributing to the discussion of such events is known as the "butterfly effect." The butterfly effect is a metaphor positing the notion that a small change in initial conditions or at some place in a complex system can have large effects on the entire system. It suggests that even a very small variance in initial conditions can make huge differences in subsequent system developments.

[1] The fact that they are self-organizing systems in no way implies that the systems will organize into optimal or even desirable system states.

A second formulation that contributes to an understanding of the dominance of uncertainty in our lives and in the outcome of policies looks at the other end of the spectrum – the mega change. This formulation is called "the black swan." A black swan "lies outside the realm of regular expectations, because nothing in the past can convincingly point to its possibility … it carries an extreme impact" (Taleb 2007, p. xvii). For example, the development of the Internet was unforeseen before its invention and has had a massive impact on society worldwide.

The fundamental lesson is that change is inevitable and that those who fail to adapt to new circumstances do so at their own peril and, unfortunately, at the peril of others. We believe hospital owners found themselves in a turbulent environment in the 1990s; their world changed fundamentally. SB 1953 appeared as the turmoil in healthcare economics emerged and became a dominant force in hospital management. Not only was the healthcare industry involved with a major transformation that created serious financial problems for most acute care hospitals, but the state and local governments were increasingly in financial difficulty. The State was verging on fiscal collapse and local governments were strained to generate sufficient revenue to cover their expected costs. The combination of these two exceptional circumstances created a context within which little money was available for retrofitting or replacing hospital facilities.

No one knows the extent to which the reactions of hospital owners to SB 1953 would have been different had hospitals been in good financial condition and had local governments had sufficient resources to address problems at hospitals they owned. Other factors such as strategy would have still affected hospital decisions. There is no doubt in our minds, though, that the economic and financial turmoil enveloping governments and hospitals seriously exacerbated both their reluctance and their inability to envision and initiate activities leading to compliance.

13.2 Adaptation in the Face of Contextual Dynamics and Unanticipated Consequences

Benjamin Disraeli is said to have noted that "Change is inevitable. Change is constant." It has been repeated so often in one way or another of late that, while true, it has become trite. Nonetheless, it is surprising to us how often that understanding is not reflected in public policy making and program administration.

We have examined how problem framing and sensemaking and environmental dynamics can affect the implementation experience. This section explores the implications of contextual dynamics, morphing problems, and unanticipated consequences on program implementation. A thread running through this discussion of obstacles to implementation is that contextual change typically creates implementation problems. Here, we address another element of change that can affect policy implementation: morphing problems.

In the face of continual change, Ashby's (1956) work on the necessity of creating means for coping with change is particularly relevant. Ashby essentially says that, in order to survive, a system must have an array of coping mechanisms at least equal to the variety of challenges it faces from its environment. In the case of SB 1953, the Law of Requisite Variety seems to cut two ways. First, the hospitals facing the need to upgrade needed coping mechanisms to deal with the regulations in SB 1953. Many of them did not have those coping mechanisms initially, nor were they able to develop them rapidly. As a consequence of being unable to cope with both existing financial difficulties and the looming costs of compliance, some hospitals failed. Others fought a delaying action while working to develop coping capabilities. A few, notably Kaiser-Permanente, with its vertically integrated structure, had adequate coping mechanisms built into their organizational design, specifically an adequate cash flow, to deal with the SB 1953 challenges. Finally, more hospitals began to integrate the legislatively mandated need to upgrade their facilities into their business strategies: if they could find the capital to build new facilities, those facilities would better meet their need for increased efficiencies and more contemporary treatment methods.

Second, the Law of Requisite Variety applies also to OSHPD and the State of California. The State's attempts at developing coping mechanisms for the problems engendered for hospitals by SB 1953 were to provide time extensions for hospitals that could qualify under the terms of specific legislation. The most significant coping mechanism adopted was the choice to essentially give hospitals classified as SPC-1 a chance to be reclassified to SPC-2 by applying the HAZUS methodology modified specifically for that application. This change in policy bought time for a significant number of hospitals that were, for the most part, simply unable to comply with the existing SB 1953 deadlines if they were to remain classified as SPC-1.

Program adaptations were made almost from the beginning of the program. Responding to both OSHPD and hospital owners, the California legislature made periodic moves to provide extensions for hospitals unable to comply with the original deadlines so that they could be in compliance with the law. Those adaptations, though welcome, were a minor and a piecemeal approach to fixing the legislation and the program.

Government bureaucracy everywhere takes a great deal of criticism from some members of the public and from some elected officials. Some of that criticism may be warranted, but certainly not in the case of OSHPD's methodological shift to employ HAZUS to evaluate hospital facilities that had been assigned SPC-1 status. Neither the legislature nor the executive branch was able to come up with a way to ease the problems associated with SB 1953 program implementation; the task was left to the administering agency and it made a bold, effective move that sidestepped the growing political conflict and the hardening of positions that was developing around SB 1953.

That having been said, it makes sense for an administering agency to monitor continually the consequences of its programs and, then, to make (or lobby for) adjustments to it based on what has been learned. It is difficult to adapt to changes in contexts and outcomes if one is unaware of them or ignores them. We know that huge changes took place in the operating environment of hospitals at about the same time SB 1953 arrived on the scene. Within that dynamic context, it was essential that some adaptations be made to adapt the SB 1953 approach and timetable to accommodate contextual change.

13.3 Morphing Problems and Adaptation

Just as contexts change, problems, too, change. Sometimes problems change because our perceptions or understanding change. Other times, problems change because conditions change. Still other times, the problem on which concern is focused gives rise to new problems that dwarf the initial problem. As problems change, they often render old views and old solutions irrelevant. Continuing to hammer away at the problem that is no longer there is generally futile and often dysfunctional. Meanwhile, any efforts to acknowledge the existence of the newly emerging problems take time and so does the development of policy to address them.

In the world of natural hazards, examples of morphing problems and problems giving rise to other problems abound. Poverty gives rise to denuding hillsides of forests. Denuded hillsides and mountains give rise to flooding, mudslides, and more poverty coupled with loss of life and destroyed villages and cities. When an Arkansas fish farmer faces a problem of too much algae in his ponds and imports Asian carp to deal with that problem, a few floods and a few years later, the Great Lakes are faced with a catastrophe of almost unthinkable proportions as the Asian carp threaten destruction of the lakes' ecosystems. When levees are built to control flooding, they open the door for extensive development in flood plains and even flood channels. When those levees fail or are overtopped, hundreds of millions of dollars in property and thousands of human and animal lives are placed in jeopardy. The list is almost endless.

Intervening in any complex system is a hazardous undertaking, even if it is only bring rabbits to Australia, mongooses to Hawaii, or starlings to North America. Even so, governments, spurred on by special interests, at least some of which have the public interest at heart, devise means for intervening in complex social and economic systems almost every day. They usually do so without benefit of competent analysis of the risks associated with that intervention and the likely consequences, both intended and unexpected. Furthermore, the risks associated with uninformed policy interventions are that the problems they are intended to address are formulated with silos of interest and responsibility. Narrowly construing problems that are integral parts of broader systems and broader concerns is undertaken too lightly too often; it is largely a consequence of how we have structured our government. That structure was perhaps adequate in a more placid, random environment. It is not adequate in a world in which is characterized by turbulent environments and tightly-coupled systems.[2] What is needed today is for problem definitions and action-oriented policies to be given much more critical thought than they have been given previously.

[2] We use the term tightly-coupled systems to describe situations in which there is little slack between interrelated systems that can absorb the consequences of uncertainty. A simple example should suffice. Just-in-time practices in manufacturing became a standard that was intended to reduce the costs of inventorying parts and material used in the manufacturing process. It works well until it doesn't. Almost-in-time is not really acceptable. Never-in-time is a lot worse. Just-in-time replaced warehousing. Warehousing was considered wholly acceptable when most goods moved by rail and when interest rates were exceptionally low. Warehousing provided the slack necessary to absorb shocks in the system. Just-in-time does not.

The assumption that a problem and the contextual dynamics enveloping it will remain constant is a recipe for disaster. Trial and error is no longer a very acceptable approach when intervening in complex situations with the likelihood of extensive, expensive repercussions.

In the case of SB 1953, we concluded that the way the "old hospital" problem was defined was so narrow that it became an obstacle to implementation. It started out as a problem defined primarily in terms of hospital facilities that were thought to be inadequate to survive a moderate earthquake and continue to function. That concern was only part of a much more complicated and tightly interwoven situation. Many hospital facilities were, indeed, subject to earthquake damage, but they were also generally obsolete or bordering on being obsolete, medical practice was changing dramatically, healthcare finance was undergoing traumatic transformation, access to affordable healthcare was diminishing, government was in serious financial condition, and alternate means for providing post-disaster care that may have been more cost-effective were not pushed. The narrow construction of the problem within that context exacerbated the larger interconnected set of problems.

The problem continued to morph as hospitals began closing, primarily in low income areas where few were insured and where the costs of service were borne by the hospitals and by state medical assistance programs. As we have said, SB 1953 may not have caused the closures, but it certainly contributed to them. The problem had been viewed originally as one in which, if the hospitals could not function following an earthquake, the injured could not be served. The problem became that fewer and fewer hospitals would be available both *before and after* the earthquake to serve existing patients and those injured in the earthquake. As one hospital executive told us, "SB 1953 may help us deal with earthquake risk, but in doing so, it puts our balance sheet at risk. How does that help anyone?"

When SB 1953 was enacted, there was a general understanding that California had too many hospital beds for the new treatment methods that were emerging. Hospital closures certainly reduced the number of surplus beds, but it reduced the number of beds primarily in low income areas. Thus, the aggregate number of beds came closer to what might be needed, but the geographical distribution of the remaining beds was far from desirable. This, coupled with the dramatic number of emergency room closures was creating serious problems of access and availability. The problem was then no longer one in which earthquake safety advocates should lead the charge, but one in which healthcare providers generally and the State government specifically should have begun to address the question of access to healthcare facilities. This has not yet happened, again in part because of the continuing revenue problems facing the State and local governments. At the same time, charitable organizations were unlikely to provide those hospital services because there was simply no way to cover the costs of operation in those circumstances, particularly when emergency rooms became the primary care physician for so many low income and uninsured people.

The basic question goes far beyond any issues associated with SB 1953. Government interventions to reduce the ability of organizations to externalize their costs and their risks to members of the public are warranted. When the consequences of decisions by, for example, a single fish farmer in Arkansas threaten the aquatic viability of the Great Lakes, then regulation is warranted. The potential for adverse consequences of thoughtless actions by a few for the many is heightened when complex systems are tightly-coupled and when the environment of those systems is densely populated by other complex systems. How, then, can we organize and structure ourselves in a generally turbulent and tightly-coupled context to be alert to problems within specialized areas and yet address those problems sensibly within the broader context, while being alert for unanticipated consequences and responding rapidly with sensible coping strategies? For us, this is the fundamental reason for attempting to understand the nexus of problem framing, policy formulation, and implementation.

References

Ashby WR (1956) Variety, constraint, and the law of requisite variety. An introduction to cybernetics. Chapman and Hall, London. See Chapter 7, pp 123–134

Baumgartner F, Jones B (2009) Agendas and instability in American politics, 2nd edn. The University of Chicago Press, Chicago

Calista D (1994) Policy implementation. In: Nagel S (ed) Encyclopedia of policy studies. Marcel Dekker, New York, pp 117–155

Emery FE,.Trist EL (1965) The causal texture of organizational environments. In: Pasmore WA,. Sherwoods JJ (eds) (1978) Sociotechnical systems: a sourcebook, University Associates, Inc., La Jolla

Sabatier PA (1986) Top-down and bottom-up approaches to implementation research: a critical analysis and suggested synthesis. J Public Pol 6:21–48

Taleb NN (2007) The black swan. Random House, New York

Part V
Putting It All Together

The authors conceptualize an "ecology of public policy implementation" that provides a frame of reference for those advocating, conceptualizing, and drafting public risk reduction policies that rely on others to spend resources to achieve the policy objectives. Just as with any complex system functioning within a complex environment, public policies focused on reducing the likely consequences of extreme events must be congruent with the systems within which they are introduced. Since risk reduction policies typically require changes in behaviors among targeted elements of the system, policymakers and program designers must have a basic understanding of the likely consequences of their intervention into that system if they expect that intervention to result in the desired outcomes.

Chapter 14
The Ecology of Public Policy Implementation

14.1 Three Questions and Some Answers

In Chap. 1, we wrote that our study of the SB 1953 experience was initiated to help us answer three questions we considered central to understanding natural hazard public policy implementation, particularly when the policy focused on regulating the behavior and investments of others.

1. What are the primary obstacles to implementing public regulatory policies intended to reduce the risks associated with hazardous events?
2. How do formal organizations make choices about how much if anything to spend to mitigate the likely consequences of rare but potential extremely destructive events?
3. What characteristics of public policies intended to reduce the risks associated with hazardous events increase the likelihood that those policies will be implemented successfully?

Some will read this book and conclude that we "took the side of the bad guys": the hospital owners whose facilities were not up to snuff in terms of seismic safety. In their view, we will have been negligent in not espousing the virtue of the cause of enhanced seismic safety. We do not see it that way. We believe strongly in the need to mitigate against the likely consequences of hazardous events and that, sometimes, it takes public regulation of private behavior to protect the public interest. We have concluded, nonetheless, that public policy that is devised without attention to congruence and context has little chance of being successful in achieving the desired ends without unnecessary adverse side effects. Thus, our efforts have been intended to assist policy makers and students of policy with understanding the obstacles they face and some means for overcoming them.

In Part 3 of the book, we focused on a topic that has not been explored extensively by students of policy implementation. Specifically, we looked at how and why the owners of acute care hospital facilities judged to not meet contemporary standards of seismic safety responded to the mandate as they did. Our more

D.J. Alesch et al., *Natural Hazard Mitigation Policy: Implementation, Organizational Choice, and Contextual Dynamics*, Environmental Hazards,
DOI 10.1007/978-94-007-2235-4_14,

encompassing objective was to gain some insight into how organizations make what we choose to call the hazard mitigation investment decision. We have not answered that question definitively. We have, though, made what we think are some significant inroads toward that answer.

First, we confirmed what many already knew: one cannot assume that organizations outside the policy making unit of government will automatically comply with directives and regulations imposed on them. Their decision of whether, how, and when to comply depends on myriad variables that the organization must consider and not on a single criterion, such as net present cost or a benefit-cost ratio. Seismic safety advocates often present choices to owners of facilities based on calculations of expected losses to earthquakes and estimated costs of taking steps that may or may not diminish or preclude those damages. From these estimates, advocates assign some net present worth to enhancing protection against seismic or other natural hazard events. We think that most organizational decision makers see those numbers as what they are: approximations of gains and losses based on assumptions having to do with estimates of the proximity, magnitude, duration, and consequences of an event that may happen at some unknown time in the future. Thus, as organizations make decisions about how to allocate scarce resources, they evaluate their choices about whether, what, and when to do something based on the assets available and on how the expenditure will contribute to a variety of objectives, only one of which is enhanced safety from a natural hazard event.

We hypothesize that, when they consider spending money on reducing the likely consequences of hazardous events, organizations are more likely than not to approach the decision more as an insurance decision than as an investment decision. That is, operating on the belief that the expenditures on "insurance" will not generate income but may save costs, they decide how much they are willing and able to spend on this form of insurance given their other priorities.

The extent to which the policy is successfully implemented depends to a very considerable extent on the response of the organizations it targets. We posited in Part 3 a set of prerequisites to organizational action with respect to circumstances with potential implications for them. We concluded that organizations must be aware that a problem exists and believe that there is something they can do about it. The organization must also believe that an acceptable solution to the problem exists and that it is in the organization's best interest to act now rather than later. Finally, it must have the wherewithal to act. If any of the prerequisites is absent, then the likelihood of organizational action is significantly reduced.

Part 4 of the book explored a second question: the obstacles to policy implementation. Most of the public policy implementation literature focuses on structure, process and the nature of participant behaviors and identifies obstacles to implementation that arise from government structures and policies and from various characteristics of the process itself or of participants in the policy implementation process. This is understandable because implementation is a critical element of policy studies and policy studies are primarily a focus of political scientists. As we noted in Chap. 1, it is entirely reasonable that "the focus of the traditional implementation and public administration literature lies mostly on governmental – or at least nominally governmentally controlled – entities. Implementation scholars are usually educated as political scientists, and as such they notice what they have been trained to see." Hill (2003) goes on to say that "by ignoring nongovernmental actors in the implementation process, scholars have overlooked important factors that shape implementation" (p. 268).

The existing literature provided us with an indispensible entrée into the implementation process. In this book, we have attempted to go beyond the focus of those studies to draw from a broader set of disciplinary perspectives to learn how they can shed light on obstacles to implementation. We concerned ourselves with problem formulation and sensemaking, organizational behavior, and organizational decision making. This approach led us to look outside the traditional focus of policy implementation research in order to identify other variables that have a significant bearing on public policy and program implementation.

Two of the areas we were led by the case study are the way in which the problems giving rise to the policy are framed and converted into policies and programs, and the characteristics of the larger context within which policy formulation and implementation takes place. In our inquiry, we concluded that the extent to which policies are implemented is affected by events that occur even before the policy is adopted. It starts with the policy itself, how the focal problem is framed and articulated, and on the means for implementation specified in the legislation. Then, implementation obstacles arise depending on the extant context within which the policy is promulgated and on the changes in the context.

The third question has to do with how it might be possible to design policy so as to overcome some of the obstacles to implementation. Our conclusions flow from our analysis. It begins with how the problem is framed and the policy options that are considered. We are not so naïve to believe for a moment that some policymakers are above manipulating problem definitions to serve their ends in other, perhaps related areas of concern. Nor do we believe that the choice of policy strategies is always the product of the best thinking or even of clear thinking. Human beings are boundedly rational.

Importantly, we do not think this was the case with SB 1953; we saw no evidence of problem manipulation or solutions selected to serve other ends. In contrast, we see well-intentioned people trying to solve a problem as they frame it. Most professional policy analysts outside of ideologically based think tanks are trained to walk around the dark crystal peering through the cloudy facets to gain the best understanding of the phenomenon under study that they can, and to think about the problem outside the constraints of narrow silos. In our experience, those organizations employ teams comprising members with diverse disciplinary expertise to help ensure that the problem is well understood. They do this before they begin to identify possible solutions to the problem or interventions in the system. Then, they create models of the system under study and identify the likely consequences of one or another intervention in it, working to identify the most approach that meets multiple criteria. Technical experts are evaluated using different criteria than members of regulatory agencies; their agenda subsequently differs. They also tend to be structured loosely, and not according to disciplinary backgrounds. We do not, of course, suggest that policy be left to technical experts; we do suggest that their skills be used to help explore the likely consequences of various decisions.

This approach works when there is sufficient common ground between interests that reasonable people can seek the best truth available and a mutually acceptable course of action. It does not work when the interests are hopelessly split by deep-seated ideological differences and partisan politics. When such splits exist, problems are defined and policies are enacted by whoever has the most votes at the moment, and that is likely to exacerbate already contentious and sometimes incendiary conditions.

We concluded, too, that the policy drafted should be congruent with the basic prerequisites to action of those organizations expected to initiate, carry out, and pay for the actions that actually result in policy implementation. When the policy is incongruent with the prerequisites to action, as we observed in the case of SB 1953, implementation problems are sure to arise.

Finally, the SB 1953 experience clearly spells out the need for government to be able to be responsive to problems like unanticipated consequences and lagging compliance that often manifest themselves during implementation. It is likely that only a few of the snags that are likely to arise once agencies begin to administer policies and programs will be identified in advance. Agencies must be alert to those emerging snags and unanticipated consequences and be encouraged to bring them to the early attention of the executive and the legislature for remedial action. In California, legislative term limits and fiscal nightmares in the State budget essentially precluded prompt response of sufficient magnitude to address the problem. Instead, numerous bills were passed that nibbled away at the edges of the problem. It took bold action on the part of the administrative agency to ease what might have been, and could still be, a policy and programmatic fiasco.

14.2 What We Mean by the Ecology of Public Policy Implementation

As we progressed through a decade or more of watching the SB 1953 experience, we had the very good fortune of not having to base our conclusions on a snapshot of the program at any one time or solely on the retrospective recollections of process participants. Instead of sequential snapshots, we were able to view the equivalent of a motion picture, viewing events and opinions in real time, writing them down, and, then, later, making sense of what we had seen. It was clear to us that we were watching much more than the "implementation process." We were watching policy making, implementation, response, and adaptation within a context that was continually changing and that had important consequences for what was happening and how the experience was unfolding. We concluded that we were studying policy implementation within its natural habitat: a dynamic environment that continually influences choices being made by those involved in all the many aspects of administering, responding, and adapting to the problem and the policy. What was happening was certainly not linear. Nor was it simply iterative; it was both interactive and stochastic. For want of a better term, we've called this more encompassing set of variables affecting policy implementation "the ecology of public policy implementation." Here, in the concluding chapter of the book, we have put what we learned from our study of the SB 1953 experience and from our analysis of what others have learned about implementation into a framework that contributes to our understanding and, we hope, to yours.

We have been slightly reluctant to use the term ecology because of its traditional application to the study of living organisms and their environment. We are emboldened to do so because the widespread use of the term human ecology has legitimized use of "ecology" to include the relationship of humans to their social, political, and economic environments. Thus, we offer no apologies.

The ecology of public policy implementation means to us the processes and the context within which policies and programs are devised and promulgated as well as the outcomes, both intended and unintended, that occur as a consequence. The ecology of public policy is not limited to the extent to which traditional implementation processes work once a policy is adopted. It begins with how the concern arises, how it is framed and articulated, the alignment of interests for and against, the bargaining or the power politics involved, the responses of targeted individuals or organizations, the contextual variables that condition and influence the response of those that are targeted, and the means available (given our bounded rationality) for fixing problems and making adaptations.

14.3 Elements of the Ecology of Public Policy Implementation

Public policy formation and implementation takes place within a set of institutions and rules, but it isn't that simple. The processes that occur within those institutions and rules are not rigid; they play out differently depending on the substantive issues and the governmental and nongovernmental actors involved. They comprise a somewhat amorphous system, often characterized by twists and turns as it proceeds, not unlike a mystery novel in which the crime is not evident, the evidence is questionable, the butler may or may not have done it, and in which the last page is hardly ever the last page. All of this takes place within a much larger environment that is often independent of the processes, but which can have a significant impact on both the process and the outcomes and which is, ultimately, affected, often in unknown ways, by the policy outcomes.

We've concluded that we can characterize the ecology of public policy implementation in terms of four basic components. These are: institutional structure and processes; substantive elements of the problem, the policy, and the programs; participatory involvement, and; contextual dynamics. These components are interrelated and influence one another.

14.3.1 Institutional Structure and Processes

As we've said, most of the literature on public policy implementation has focused on what goes on within governments and between governments and governmental agencies. Without doubt, these are a main component of the ecology of public policy implementation. How we structure the executive and legislative branches of government makes a difference on how we conceptualize problems and solutions, particularly because of the silos into which they are organized. The rules that govern the processes involved in policy formulation and the development of regulations with the force of law not only make the processes (if not the outcomes) relatively predictable and, in many ways, uniform, but can also contribute to or thwart policy development and implementation.

The array of government agencies involved in program implementation and the levels at which they exist are part of the structure and processes component. So, too, are those who work in program administration and make choices every day about what to do, how to do it, and how to address the myriad of issues and questions that arise each day without benefit of a pre-programmed response. In the case of SB 1953, policy formation and implementation took place within only one level of government, but a number of agencies were involved in a variety of ways.

14.3.2 Substantive Elements of the Problem

A second component of the ecology of public policy implementation consists of the substantive elements of the problem that is the focus of the governmental institutions and organizations within which policymaking and implementation occur. The problem being addressed may be procedural or substantive or it may be a substantive concern disguised as a procedural issue. The nature and the substance of a problem define the interests that are aroused and, hence, the players that come forward to attempt to influence the outcomes of the processes. The substance of the problem and the solutions proposed or adopted may have trivial or major consequences for the social, economic, and political system within which the policy makers live and it may have consequences for other such systems as well. One important characteristic of the substantive elements of the problem is the extent to which the policy has or is likely to have significant intended or unintended consequences.

The characteristics of a problem or a candidate public problem have implications for policy making concerning it and for implementation. Decades ago, Platt (1969) published a useful list of criteria for characterizing problems. Paraphrasing his list, we can characterize problems in terms for whom it is a problem, how many or how much is at risk, the nature and level of the consequences that are expected unless action is taken, where and the kinds of places in which it is to occur, and the urgency of addressing the problem. One would expect that the more consequential the problem, the more likely it is to involve controversy, partisan politics, and divergent interest groups.

One other characteristic of a problem or candidate problem is likely to affect the policymaking and program development process and the outcomes of that process. Problems that appear to be complex, difficult, or intractable pose particular challenges to policymakers. March and Olsen (1973) take the position that, many times, no one actually attempts to resolve the problem at hand. They maintain that decision makers may ignore the problem or defer considering it, convert the problem into another problem more easily dealt with, or, rarely, actually resolve the problem. Fioretti (2009), in his agent-based models testing the original formulation, adds "buck-passing" as a fourth option employed by decision and policy makers. One variation of policy making strategies includes approaching extremely difficult problems by construing them as problems that are narrower in nature. A second variation is to frame or disguise one problem as another: illustratively, a governor's attempt to weaken state and local government employee unions may be framed instead as an effort to balance a temporary budget deficit.

The substance of a public problem or candidate public problem and the strategies employed by advocates to have it enacted as policy and by opponents to preclude or to modify the policy have a decided effect on the policy, the programs intended to implement it, and the subsequent consequences.

14.3.3 Participatory Involvement

The parties involved in policy making and implementation include those who frame the problem, those who form and enact the policy, those who administer the program, and those who are expected to take the actions that actually achieve the desired outcomes, regardless of whether they are part of the policymaking government. The literature indicates that actors at each "stop" in the process influence, to a greater or lesser extent, influence policy, implementation, and policy outcomes. The literature further indicates that their implementation activities may have either a positive or adverse effect on outcomes. Our analysis of the SB 1953 experience demonstrates the extent to which actions by organizations targeted in the policy can affect implementation outcomes.

Large numbers of policies and programs are adopted at all levels of government and pass "under the radar." They are a matter of concern to a small number of parties, may deal with minor matters, do not warrant attention in the media, and are fully implemented by public officials. Other policy discussions make headlines and involve large numbers of sometimes vociferous and contentious actors representing a disparate set of interests. Some of the participants are, of course, required to be involved since they are authoritative and legitimate policy makers. Some are administrative agencies. Others represent special interests and points of view, such as labor representatives, seismic safety advocates, building owners, and others. Motivation for involvement varies considerably. For some, it is a core concern; for others it is only one among many issues. Some organizations are almost always present when specific kinds of issues arise; others join in from time to time as issues become particularly salient or otherwise useful to them.

14.3.4 Contextual Dynamics

The fourth component in the ecology of public policy implementation is the context within which the process takes place. In Chap. 12 we examined the influence of the broader, dynamic context on program implementation and outcomes. That context exists and changes largely independently from the policy implementation activities, but the nature of the context can be affected by implementation activities. Illustratively, the increasing cost of structural steel and concrete in California during the 1990s affected the costs of complying with SB 1953, but as hospital construction increased, that construction exacerbated the cost of structural steel and concrete. The context changes continually, usually at the margins, but sometimes episodically, rapidly and dramatically.

14.4 Concluding Comment

As the population and the wealth of the United States continue to be concentrated in the parts of the nation that are most subject to hazardous events from nature and from humans, it is imperative that much more attention be given to hazard mitigation. We have the technical knowledge but not the political will to reduce the adverse consequences of the earthquakes, hurricanes, floods, storm surges, volcanic eruptions, and other events that are certain to occur. We are much more willing to pick up the pieces and bury the dead following a hazardous event and then struggle to achieve aggregate community recovery and what the Japanese have come to call "life recovery" than we are to use sensible means to prevent the economic losses and the social and personal costs that are the consequences of hazardous events. Back in 1999, we took on this case study, which has occupied us on and off for more than a decade, in the hope that we could identify the primary obstacles to hazard mitigation and, based on that, provide counsel to those who advocate such mitigation can on how to pursue that end more effectively.

References

Fioretti G (2009) Passing the buck in the garbage can model of organizational choice. Unpublished. Online at http://mpra.ub.uni-muenchen.de/16977/. MPRA paper no. 16977, posted 27 Aug 2009

Hill HC (2003) Understanding implementation: street-level bureaucrats' resources for reform. J Public Admin Theor 13(3):265–282

March JG, Olsen JP (1973) Ambiguity and choice in organizations. Universitetsforlaget Bergen, Norway

Platt J (1969) What we must do. Science 166(3909):1115–1121, November 28

Index

D.J. Alesch et al., *Natural Hazard Mitigation Policy: Implementation, Organizational Choice, and Contextual Dynamics*, Environmental Hazards, DOI 10.1007/978-94-007-2235-4,

MIX
Papier aus verantwortungsvollen Quellen
Paper from responsible sources
FSC® C105338

If you have any concerns about our products,
you can contact us on
ProductSafety@springernature.com

In case Publisher is established outside the EU,
the EU authorized representative is:
Springer Nature Customer Service Center GmbH
Europaplatz 3, 69115 Heidelberg, Germany

Printed by Libri Plureos GmbH
in Hamburg, Germany